The
Parent
Guidebook

Also by Mary B. Seger, NP, PhD

Books

Invite Joy Into Your Life: Steps For Women Who Want to Rediscover the Simple Pleasures of Living

e-Newsletter

Mary's Musings

Miscellaneous

Joy! Cards

Finding Your Joy: A Journal

All of these items are available at **www.maryseger.com**

The
Parent
Guidebook

How to raise happy, healthy children
with advice from
a mom and nurse practitioner

Author of *Invite Joy Into Your Life*
Mary B. Seger, NP, PhD

Sophia Rose
Press

www.maryseger.com

Seger, Mary B.
   The parent guidebook : how to raise happy, healthy children with advice from a mom and nurse practitioner / Mary B. Seger. — Gaylord, Mich. : Sophia Rose Press, c2012.

   p. ; cm.

   ISBN: 978-0-9790461-3-1

   Includes bibliographical references and index.

   Summary: The guidelines in this book help readers with the basics of child rearing from infancy to adulthood, aiming to make life less stressful. Also includes guidelines for pregnancy, postpartum drepression, diseases related to diet, the truth about certain foods, healthy eating tips and recommended supplements, and provides recipes.—Publisher.

   1. Child rearing. 2. Parenting. 3. Parent and child. 4. Children—Nutrition. 5. Pregnancy. 6. Postpartum depression. I. Title.

HQ769 .S44 2012   2012902468
649/.1—dc23   1204

Printed in the United States of America

Design by Mary Jo Zazueta / www.tothepointsolutions.com

To My Roses:

Grandma, Stephanie, and Amelia

Contents

Introduction

"Mom, I'm pregnant," said my daughter, Stephanie, over the phone.

How can you be pregnant? I thought. *I am still getting used to the fact you are an adult. I remember when you were getting ready to leave for college and I panicked, thinking of all the things I had not yet taught you. And now . . . a baby?*

There is so much information I want to pass on, things I learned and knowledge others shared with me. *Where do I begin?* As I sit, contemplating (and panicking), many thoughts come to mind. I grab a piece of paper and a pen and start to write. I think about my pregnancy and what I experienced along the way . . .

I am amazed at how fast twenty years has flown by. I remember Stephanie as a toddler in the toy store and her cry of "Baby!" when she saw a beautiful doll. We had to get it for her. Oh, how she mothered her doll. Stephanie played in her pretend kitchen and cooked food for her baby. Her greatest joy was reading books to her baby. And when she was a teenager, I watched how gentle, loving, and yet firm she was with little ones. In what seems like the blink of an eye, my daughter has matured into a strong, independent, wise, and loving young woman.

I also remember having postpartum depression, which is on the rise. I have included information on the causes of and measures you can take to help with this common yet oftentimes hidden ailment.

As I look at my notes, I am pleased. They are the basic guidelines for parenting, short and easy to read. As any young mother knows, there is little time to do much of anything except take care of the baby.

As Stephanie approached the birth of her baby and becoming a mother, I asked what she thought I had done right as a mother. She said:

★ Teaching me to take care of myself and be responsible at a young age

★ How to help around the house

★ Teaching me discipline so I wasn't a brat and I learned to appreciate things from you

★ Finding the balance between being a mother and friendship

★ Hanging out and having fun together

Whew! It is nice to know I got it right some of the time.

I am a nurse practitioner with a PhD in Natural Health. I have an integrative medicine practice in internal medicine and women's healthcare. My focus is on diet, exercise, stress reduction, herbs and supplements, along with traditional medical care. I decided this would be the perfect forum for sharing what I have learned and experienced, as a mother and a professional.

Your children will cause you to feel every emotion imaginable, from the greatest love and joy to the deepest despair, depression, and, at times, rage.

Good luck and enjoy!

Stephanie Rose

Stephanie, my sweet pea
Soon, a mother to be
How can this be?
My baby, a grown woman
Bringing Amelia Rose into being
The miracle of life

So quick, so fast, in the blink of an eye
I go from holding my baby
To see my daughter hold hers

My daughter, my granddaughter
Tears well in my eyes
My heart over flows with love
Two miracles before me
Thank you! Thank you! Thank you!

~ Mary B Seger

The
Parent
Guidebook

Guidelines for Child Rearing

Guideline: a general rule, principle, or piece
of advice

Child Rearing: the act of training or bringing
up a child; the interaction
between parent and child

1

If mama ain't happy, nobody's happy.

You will find when you have a bad day, your child will, too. On the flipside, if mama is happy, so is everyone else. If you are having a series of bad days, it would benefit you to assess the situation. Sometimes it helps to discuss your life with someone who has words of wisdom. Most women need to talk it out, to figure it out. Ask yourself, "What will it take to make me happy?"

Insanity is doing the same thing over and over again and expecting different results.
~ Albert Einstein

You are responsible for your happiness. Waiting for someone to change so you can be happy is a waste of time and will not lead you down a path of joy. If you are not happy with the results you are currently getting, make a change. Make different choices. A change might upset some people, but remember: If mama ain't happy, nobody's happy!

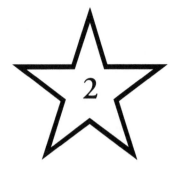

Stop. Look. Listen.

Take time to see the wonder and magic of the world through the eyes of your child.

**Do not torture yourself or
others by taking your infant
or toddler to a restaurant
that is not child friendly.**

Hire a baby-sitter or order take-out.

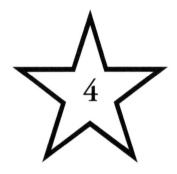

Slow down. You will never get everything done.

Pick one to three tasks to accomplish each day. Celebrate what you finish instead of berating yourself for what you do not.

One of my patients discussed her lack of motivation to do things and wondered if she was suffering from depression. "What don't you want to do?" I asked.

"I have two bathrooms that are dirty. After I get home from work, I don't feel like cleaning them."

I laughed. "Of course, you don't. Who wants to work all day and then go home and clean bathrooms? I have found after working all day, I need to break down the household chores into smaller tasks. It takes longer but eventually everything gets done. Tonight, clean the toilets; then do something you want to do," I suggested. "Tomorrow, clean the sinks; then do something fun. In two days, do the floors, and have more fun."

"I can do that!" she said.

Make a master list of everything that needs to be done. On a cute notepad, write down one, two or three tasks for each day. Once you have completed a task, cross it off the list and the notepad. You will find some things will never get done; so cross them off the master list for good.

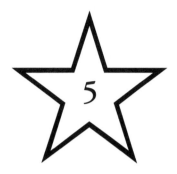

All children should eat a pound of dirt before they are three years old.

The Hygiene Hypothesis suggests exposure to allergens in one's environment early in life reduces the risk of developing allergies by boosting a person's immune system activity. When we do not expose our children to bugs and dirt at a very young age, we can prevent their immune systems from developing fully and completely. This "aversion to dirt" has resulted in an increase in allergic/atopic diseases such as asthma, allergies and dermatitis. It is also suggested that a poor immune system has an impact on autoimmune diseases, inflammatory bowel disease, and depression.

A study showed children raised in hygienic environments had higher C Reactive Protein (CRP) levels than children who were allowed normal exposure to dirt. An increased CRP in the blood is an indication of inflammation and a risk factor for heart disease.

Let go of the fear bugs and dirt will cause your children great harm. They won't. What they will do is stimulate young bodies to build strong and functional immune systems.

Teach your children good hand-washing with soap and water, especially before meals and after using the restroom. Consider avoiding the hand sanitizers in favor of soap and water. Studies have shown hand sanitizers are not effective against C difficile, a bacterium that causes diarrhea. The incidence of C difficile infections has increased dramatically, especially in the elderly and children.

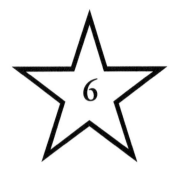

Rest on the twelfth day after giving birth.

This is an old wives' tale I heard from my Grandma Rose. I do not know of any medical reasons for this. I suspect it is simply the mother's hormones have crashed, sleep deprivation has caught up, and the realization of major life changes has sunk in.

I can report, I did not rest on the twelfth day. Instead I entertained my in-laws. Bad idea. At the end of the day, I collapsed on the couch and could not stop crying.

A day of rest is a good thing. Mark day twelve on your calendar and put your feet up.

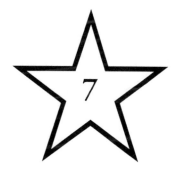

Get rid of the books and use your common sense.

As a new mother, I read everything I could get my hands on. The problem was everyone had a different opinion. I was a confused mess. In great distress, I sat down with my Aunt Jeanne and grandma to discuss all of the different opinions on what a child should be doing and at what age. Aunt Jeanne spoke these words of wisdom: "Get rid of the books and use your own common sense."

This powerful advice was incredibly helpful to me because Stephanie, my darling girl, did not, has not, and probably never will follow the typical path. (Although I think she is the most amazing young woman.)

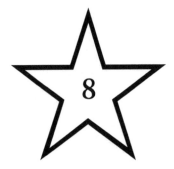

Schedules and routine are good.

Children feel secure when they know what to expect, even though they will sometimes fight the rules.

9

Give up
keeping a clean house.

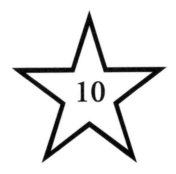

Do not use "I am going to count to three."

You are training your child to wait until you count to three.

The first time I heard this truth, I was shocked, then angry, and then I laughed. I realized children are smart and will push parents to the limit. The next time I told Stephanie to do something and she, of course, did not do it, I went after her.

She yelled, "Hey! You didn't count to three."

I said, "Hey, I am not going to count to three anymore. I want you to do what I tell you to do *when* I tell you to do it!"

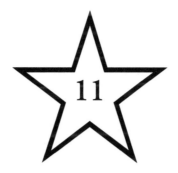

You may have to supplement the breast milk or formula sooner than you were told.

After eight weeks of interrupted sleep, I was exhausted. I called my friend Penny. "She won't sleep!" I cried.

"Feed her some rice cereal," Penny said.

"I am not supposed to feed her food yet," I blubbered.

Penny replied, "Feed her. She's starving."

I still remember trying to get the rice cereal into Stephanie's mouth with a baby spoon. She slept the night through. I woke up the next morning in a panic. I thought she had died and I had killed her. She hadn't, and I didn't.

I fed her rice cereal every night and she slept like, well, she slept like a baby! So did I.

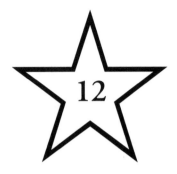

You are not Superwoman.

Take care of yourself. You cannot be all, do all, or fix all. Rip the "S" off your shirt and stop trying to be Superwoman. Stop multitasking. Do one thing at a time and then move on to the next. When you multitask, your full attention is never on any one thing and you miss out.

Look at your life. How many activities are your children and you involved in? Is the amount conducive to a sane lifestyle?

Be the human being you were born to be. Stop trying to be the perfect mother, spouse, daughter, sister, career woman, and volunteer. It is impossible. Focus on your priorities. Let go of the unimportant stuff. Trying to do it all is exhausting and will make you feel like the wicked witch of the west.

13

Don't take away the blankey or stuffed animal too soon.

In this crazy world, a little security is a good thing. Stephanie loved her blankey. She would rub the silk edging between her thumb and first two fingers. I remember wondering what this was all about. One day, with my girlfriends, I grabbed a blanket and we rubbed the silk. It was very soothing. I understood.

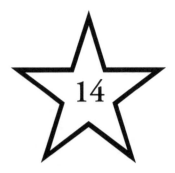

14

If your child is throwing a
fit, do not be afraid or too
embarrassed to leave the
store or restaurant.

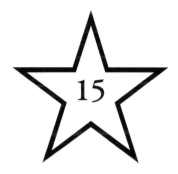

Remember, you are a parent, not your child's friend.

"If you have never been hated by your child you have never been a parent."
~Bette Davis

Maintain your role as a mother. You can be nice without acting like your child's friend, especially as she gets older. Tough love is easier when kids are in their teens than when they are in their twenties or thirties.

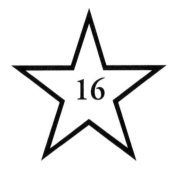

Probiotics are an effective treatment for colic.

A healthy gut is a good thing. I wish I had known this when Stephanie was a baby. She had colic and nothing I tried alleviated her discomfort, except when I lay her over my arm with my hand supporting her stomach and swung her from side to side.

Probiotics may also be helpful when treating other conditions and illnesses. See page 106 for more information.

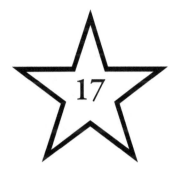

Your children will experience life differently than you.

They will do things differently . . . and that is okay.

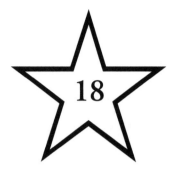

Let your children make mistakes and come up with solutions.

This is how they learn and gain self-confidence.

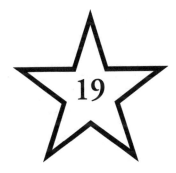

Chamomile drops soothe teething pain.

After using large amounts of acetaminophen and Orajel, I decided to find a natural treatment to ease the discomfort of teething. I was amazed by the effectiveness of Chamomile homeopathic drops (Boiron Camilia Teething Remedy).

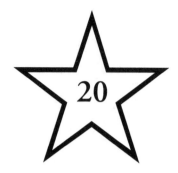

20

If your baby won't stop crying, cover her shoulders.

One day Stephanie was crying nonstop. I fed her, held her, changed her, and burped her. Nothing helped. I put her in the bassinet and called Grandma. "She won't stop crying!" I said.

"Did you cover her shoulders?" Grandma asked.

Huh? No, I had not. I covered Stephanie's shoulders with a blanket; she stopped crying and fell asleep.

(I have since discovered when I've had a bad day, covering my shoulders with a prayer shawl brings great comfort. Try it.)

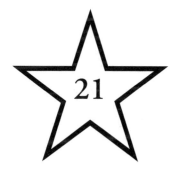

21

There may be times, due to fatigue and frustration, when you will have thoughts of harming your child.

This will scare you but know it is normal. Immediately put your baby in a safe place, and

- Take a time-out
- Eat an apple
- Call a friend
- Dance
- Do ten jumping jacks
- Take a deep breath or two or three
- Blow bubbles
- Sing loudly to a song
- Hug a pillow
- Cry

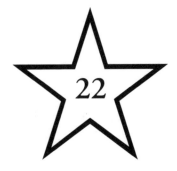

Time-outs are good for children *and* moms.

There will be moments when a break is needed, quiet time to chill. The recommendation for time-outs is to use the age of the child or the mom. For example, five minutes for a five-year-old with an attitude and twenty-five minutes for a twenty-five-year old who is feeling crabby or witchy.

If your children are older, tell them you have been a bad girl and need a time-out. This will confuse them. Enjoy!

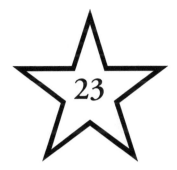

23

When rules are broken, there must be consequences.

Teach your children there are always consequences for their behavior, good *and* bad.

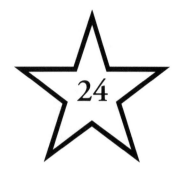

24

Give good hugs.

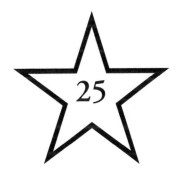

Turn off the TV.

Plan activities to do with your child:

★ Read ★ Cook ★ Play board games

★ Build a snowman ★ Make snow angels

★ Roast marshmallows ★ Walk in the woods

★ Go to the beach ★ Build sandcastles

★ Play in the leaves ★ Watch the clouds float by

★ Blow bubbles ★ Plant flowers or vegetables

★ Color ★ Dance ★ Play make-believe

★ Ride a bike ★ Swim ★ Fly a kite

★ Catch snowflakes on your tongue

★ Pack a picnic and go on an adventure

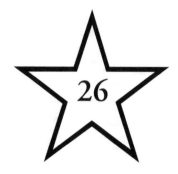

Say I love you and feel it.

Appreciate your child being a part of your life. Let love fill your heart and radiate from you to surround your child with warmth.

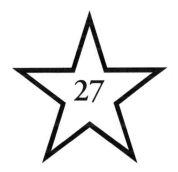

27

**Snuggle and read a
bedtime story every night.**

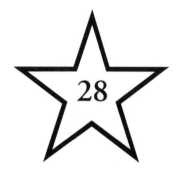

28

Choose your battles wisely.

My darling daughter was always strong-willed. One of the first battles I remember with Stephanie was over socks. When she was three years old, I purchased a bag of white socks. I was very excited. They would be easy to sort and would go with any outfit. Miss Stephanie thought otherwise and had a major meltdown. She wanted colored socks to match her outfits. After several deep breaths, I decided to give the white socks to her cousins and to shop for colored socks. This was not a battle that was important to me. Health, safety, and nutrition, yes. Not socks.

I was reminded of this story recently when a young woman came into my office for her annual exam. She told me her socks did not match and she wanted me to know it was intentional. "My mother never matched our socks and I have continued the tradition," she said.

I was impressed by this incredible time management technique. How many hours have you spent matching socks or trying to find the mate to a sock? Think of the time you would save and the frustration you would avoid. There are now companies that sell mismatched socks. It is time we bucked tradition. (My patient's mother was way ahead of her time.)

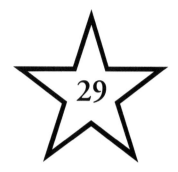

Listen to your child.

You have two ears and one mouth for a reason.

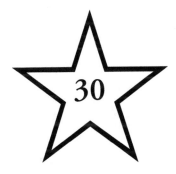

30

Teach the art of conversation.

Ask your children how their day went and let them tell you, without feeling the need to fix or criticize their stories. Insist on eye contact.

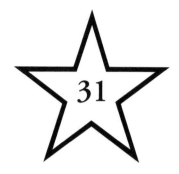

Refrain from
giving your opinion.

This can be difficult. If your child asks for your opinion, you have two options: You can give it or you can ask questions so she forms her own opinion. For example, ask her to look at an area of her life where she has made good decisions. Can she use a similar technique for this situation? Another approach is to say, "If your best friend was going through this situation, what would you tell her to do?" Then suggest your child take her own good advice.

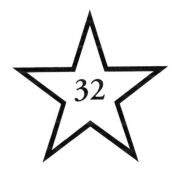

32

Use lavender essential oil to calm the arsenic hour.

The arsenic hour is when children become crabby and fussy, usually in the late afternoon and early evening. For babies younger than one, light an oil burner and place a drop of lavender essential oil in the water. When your child is one or older, put a couple drops of lavender essential oil in the bath water. Breathe deep. Ahhhh . . . This is good for mama and baby.

Do not use perfume oils. For more information on lavender essential oil go to page 111.

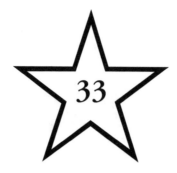

Seek other moms.

They know what you are experiencing. It helps to talk things out. There is nothing more soothing to my soul than hearing a wise and compassionate female friend say, "I know what you are going through. It will all work out okay." Especially if they have walked in my shoes.

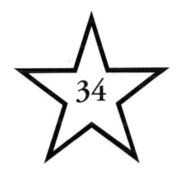

Don't say, "My child would never do that!"

She won't. She will do it twice as badly.

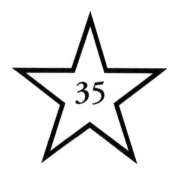

35

Honor yourself by taking time for you.

If you feel empty because all you do is give, your children will sense this and want more of you. Stop giving and take a time-out for you.

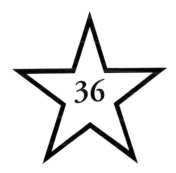

Eat at least
one meal together each day.

Turn off the TV. No reading allowed. Simply dine and converse.

Family mealtimes have been associated with healthier meals, decreased eating disorders in females, and decreased use of tobacco, alcohol, and marijuana in both males and females. A study also found children who had regular family mealtimes ate healthier as adults.

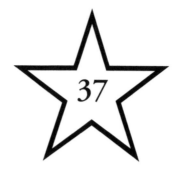

37

Teach your children manners.

★ Say please, thank you, and excuse me.

★ No passing gas, burping, or farting in public.

★ Cover your mouth when you cough or sneeze.

★ Wash hands after using the restroom and before meals.

★ No staring or pointing.

★ No swearing.

★ Write thank-you notes.

★ Open doors for others.

★ Dress appropriately for the situation.

★ Do unto others as you would have them do unto you

First impressions are a constant in society.
However, their product, the period that proves or
disproves their validity is not:
Good ones are pleasant and long-lasting; bad ones
long and difficult to disprove.
-Diego Valasquez

Why teach manners? Think about someone you met or saw and what your first impression was, good or bad. Over time the impression may have changed. Be amazed how quickly you made the decision. *Blink* by Malcolm Gladwell is a book about how people make decisions without thinking and how we make choices in the blink of an eye. Having good manners and following the social graces will always provide more opportunities for your children and yourself. Over a lifetime they will open doors that may otherwise close due to poor manners. If you do not teach your children manners, they may not know they are not following proper etiquette. I can tell you, they will be judged and not included. Don't let this happen to your children.

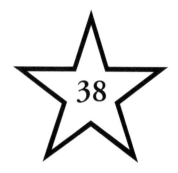

Teach children to respect their elders and how to make a proper introduction.

Shake hands firmly but don't squeeze too hard. Introduce adults by using Dr., Mr., Mrs., or Ms.

Introducing people to each other is a skill at which I am completely inept. This makes me feel awkward in social settings. I have told my husband if I don't introduce him he should introduce himself as I have completely forgotten the person's name.

I strongly suggest teaching your children how to introduce people properly as this has caused me much distress over my lifetime. As I write this, I wonder why I never learned this social grace as my mother was very strict when it came to manners. I believe it was because I grew up in a small town where we already knew everyone; so occasions for introductions were rare. As children, we were taught to address adults as Dr. Mr., Mrs. or Miss; we didn't have Ms. back then. I was also rather shy, so by the time I talked to a new person, everyone else already knew them.

As an adult, I was always impressed by my neighbor who gave excellent introductions. "Mary," she would say, "I would like you to meet Sophia Smith. Sophia, this is Mary Seger." She did it with such ease and grace. I, on the other hand, when faced with introducing someone, go into a mild panic which clears all thought from my head. Thus, my saving grace is telling my husband he is on his own. Don't let your children experience this.

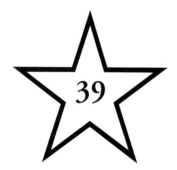

Teach proper table manners and dining etiquette.

Parents must model this behavior!

★ Do not interrupt when someone is speaking.

★ Set the table correctly.

★ Know how to use eating utensils.

★ Chew with your mouth closed.

★ Sit up to the table; no slouching.

★ No double dipping.

★ Keep your elbows and forearms off the table.

★ Put the napkin in your lap when you sit down at the table.

★ Wait until everyone is seated and served before starting to eat.

★ Slow down and savor your food; don't shovel it in.

★ No negative comments about what is being served.

★ At the end of the meal, thank the cook.

Good table manners are imperative if your children plan on being in social situations for pleasure or work. I have listed the basics above. If you are not sure if your manners are appropriate observe what other people are doing. You can also purchase a book to educate yourself and begin teaching your children. There is nothing worse than feeling awkward in a social setting. Teach children when they are young so they can enter into this world more confidently.

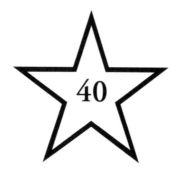

40

Have a conversation with your child before you walk into the store.

It goes like this: "I am not buying you anything today" or "When I am done with my shopping, you may pick one item costing no more than x." Be very specific and I promise your shopping excursion will go easier.

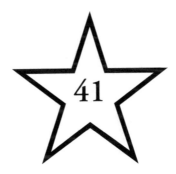

Be kind and gentle.

Offer tenderness during the rough patches of life.

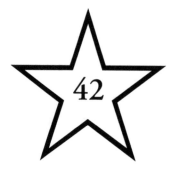

42

Sometimes you need to bite your tongue.

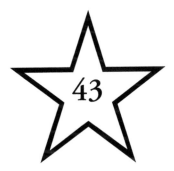

**Try to be consistent
as much as possible.**

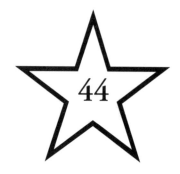

Start traditions.

Sit down and reflect on your childhood. How did you celebrate birthdays? Holidays? Vacations? Consider the traditions you would like to continue with your children. What did you enjoy? What drove you crazy? Are there any new traditions you would like to start?

I always think about my late parents during the Christmas season, all the beautiful childhood memories they worked so hard to create for their children. I can't remember a single wrapped gift that I received as a child, but I treasure in my heart the memories of our family spending evenings together in our living room, the Christmas tree lit with those big fat lights full of beautiful color. So much love, security and peace. That's a gift I get to carry in my heart and unwrap over and over again!
–Patricia Serwach

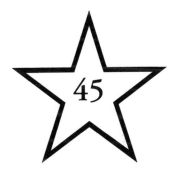

Babies change their behavior every three months . . .

then it will be every six months. You will just get your child figured out and she will change.

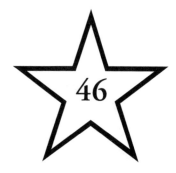

46

Do not force potty training.

I decided it was time to potty train my daughter. I got the cute potty seat, pull-ups, and offered every bribe I could think of. As time went on, with no interest on Stephanie's part, I became annoyed. Then she started to have loose stools. I took her to the pediatrician who told me Stephanie was holding her stool and to stop potty training her. She would potty train when she was ready. To let go of this took effort on my part. I told myself, "I know she will be potty trained before she goes to kindergarten." She was. When she was ready, she was ready. Pushing her only made me miserable.

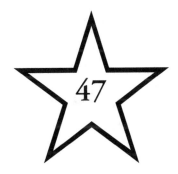

47

If your child throws a tantrum, make sure she is in a safe place and then walk away.

I still remember the day I learned this technique. Children throw tantrums for attention. My darling girl was throwing a major tantrum in the middle of the living room. I was starting to get wound up; then I remembered this advice and walked away. As I peeked in, I watched her continue for a minute, then stop, lift her head to look around for someone to witness her tantrum. No one was there. The outburst ceased. I tried not to laugh out loud.

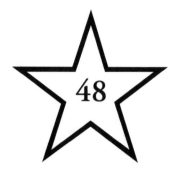

48

When training your child in a new behavior, it may take up to a week of torture before she accepts and embraces it.

When trying to change behavior or habit, you will probably meet with strong resistance. Keep calm and carry on. Do not give up. Persevere. You will be glad you did.

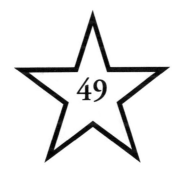

49

**Your child is watching
you, and she will
mimic what you do.**

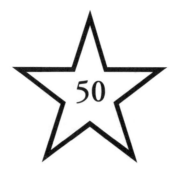

Be your child's champion.

Believe in your child. According to *Random House Thesaurus*, "champion" means to fight for, stand up for, advocate.

To be a true champion is to believe in the essence of your child. It is letting go of ego and judgment and providing support in the direction your child has chosen to take. It is doing so with an open heart.

When you believe in the cause, this can be easy. With children, however, you may not agree with the direction they are taking. At times like these, it is best to bite your tongue and keep your mouth shut. Reflect on why this is affecting you in a negative way. Remember you are in charge of your life and your perception of the events in this world, not anyone else's life. When you hear yourself say, "Well, I wouldn't have done it like that," it is time for *you* to come to peace with the situation.

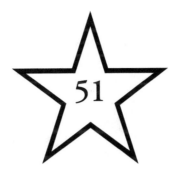

Eat healthy meals and supplement as suggested.

Feed yourself and your family a diet of protein, lots of veggies, fruit, and small amounts of grains. White flour and sugar promote insulin resistance, which can lead to heart disease, diabetes, cancer, fatty liver disease and Alzheimer's disease. If we don't stop feeding our children the Standard American Diet (SAD) they will die before we do.

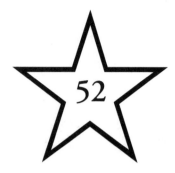

Teach your children how to swallow pills.

Swallowing pills is a critical skill. I have some patients who never learned this and it is always a challenge to find liquid medication or supplements they can take.

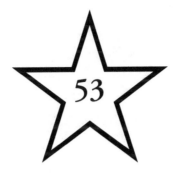

53

Time is the most precious gift you can give your child.

In the end, it is not the money or the gifts. Give your children your time and attention. It is invaluable.

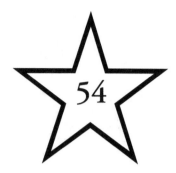

Maintain your marriage.

Marriage is like a plant. If a plant is not watered or fed it will die. Likewise, no attention paid to your marriage can cause it to fade into nonexistence.

Babies and children place stress on a marriage because the added responsibility leaves little time for your spouse. To keep your marriage alive, connect with your partner for at least ten minutes every day. You talk for five minutes; he talks for five minutes. And, at least twice a month go on a date with your husband.

These activities will allow you and your husband to communicate as adults on a regular basis. It can even increase your libido, which sometimes lessens after having children. (Ask your husband to pick up the baby-sitter and feed the kids while you get ready for the big date.)

When you spend time together as a couple, you are

setting a great example for your children. Your daughters-in-law will love you because your son learned to take his wife out on a date. Daughters will develop an expectation of spending time with their husbands.

Most importantly, when your children become teenagers or leave home, you won't be asking "Who is this man sleeping in my bed?"

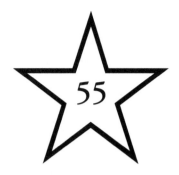

55

Make love with your husband.

Men think about sex a lot; many women don't think about sex at all, especially new mothers. Men and women are different. Go figure.

Low libido is a common complaint of women of all ages. When a woman is approached by her man to make love, there are five questions that will go through her head, each of which must be answered in a positive way or she will say, "No thanks." The questions are: Will it hurt? Am I happy with my physical appearance? Am I happy with my husband? Am I tired? Will it be fun?

If it hurts, you may need more foreplay. If that doesn't do the trick, see your healthcare provider.

If it doesn't feel good, you aren't doing it right.
~ Elaine Hammerschlag

Are you happy with your looks? Your husband just wants to make love. Get over yourself or do something about it.

> *When did you ever have a man say no when you were standing there naked?*
> Julia Roberts in the movie *Eat, Pray, Love*

Are you happy with your husband? Women must connect with their partner in order to make love. Men cannot read minds. Women are the makers of relationships. Tell him what you want or seek counseling.

Are you tired? Find a time when you are not, maybe after your date?

Is it fun? Most women tell me making love is fun once they get started. Remember this or find new ways to make it fun.

> *There is no such thing as a frigid woman, only a clumsy man.*
> ~ Virginia Kelly

Pregnancy

Before you were conceived, I wanted you
Before you were born, I loved you
Before you were here an hour, I would die for you
This is the miracle of love

~ Maureen Hawkins

When I was pregnant, my brother's girlfriend, a young woman from Japan, was shocked when she heard I was attending college. She said in Japan women rested during their pregnancies. I thought that was odd. In the U.S. when you are pregnant you just keep going, no big deal.

As I look back twenty years later, my heart is saddened. I missed it. I missed the miracle of my daughter growing inside my body. I didn't even realize I was pregnant until I was three months along. There was no time! I was in my second year of grad school, and I had complications which carried me through the sixth month.

> *How might your life have been different,*
> *if through the years, there has been a place where*
> *you could go?*
> *A place of women, who knew the cycles of life,*
> *the ebb and flow of nature,*
> *Who knew of times of work and times of quiet ...*
> *Who understood your tiredness*
> *and need for rest ...*

~ Judith Duerk, *Circle of Stones: Women's Journey to Herself*

Stephanie had a healthy pregnancy. She enjoyed it, but worked at a physically demanding job until five weeks before she delivered. Shortly before she quit working, she experienced severe cramping and finally went to the Emergency Room. She was diagnosed with a vaginal and urinary tract infection. When she went to the pharmacy to get the medication, the pharmacist said her insurance card did not go through. On her way to work, she called me, crying. At work, they told her to go home. She called her insurance company, they phoned the pharmacy, and she finally got the medication and went home to rest. To rest . . .

I realized I was not very supportive in honoring the miracle of growing a baby and the need for rest during pregnancy. Too few women in our society honor the need for rest. We keep on going until we crash, burn, and get sick. I see this daily in my practice.

"Can you go home and rest?" I ask.

"No, I have to . . ." they reply.

"If your best friend felt like you do, what would you tell her to do?" I ask.

Most times, with tears falling, these exhausted women reply, "I'd tell her to go home and rest."

Be aware of the females in your life. Be one of the women Judith Duerk describes, a woman who is aware of the need for quiet ... who understood tiredness and the need for rest. How can you be this woman to yourself and honor yourself during this time of growing a baby?

Rest and revel in the miracle of your pregnancy.

BRAIN LOSS

My husband, Bill, was telling me about his pregnant daughter, Nickie, forgetting to do something. Stephanie was also forgetting things. "It is the brain loss that occurs during pregnancy," I told him.

I remembered as my pregnancy progressed, I seemed to lose more of my brain function. I came up with an explanation, which has not been proven scientifically. I do believe any woman who has been pregnant will agree it is true. When a woman is pregnant, a hollow tube develops between her brain and the baby's brain. During the course of the pregnancy, brain matter flows from the mother to the baby. The mother is not losing her brains; rather she is giving it to her baby. This occurs with each pregnancy. The more children you have, the more brain loss. There is no reversal of this phenomenon; once you lose it, it is gone.

After Stephanie was born, I found sticky notes with the Scarecrow from *The Wizard of Oz* and the words "If I only had a brain." I sent notes to my pregnant friends with the story about brain loss so they would understand this was a normal part of pregnancy.

A BIRTH PLAN

The other night, as I listened to a webinar, a woman shared she did not feel like a real woman because she delivered her baby by C-Section. This made me sad. Let me tell you a medical fact: There are no guarantees on what will occur during labor and delivery. You can make the perfect birth plan. It may go accordingly to plan or it may not. To be attached to a birth plan is to set yourself up for frustration and disappointment.

When I had Stephanie, the only plan I had was to check my modesty at the door of the OB department. That is what the nurses I worked with told me as they knew I was very modest. On the day Stephanie was born, I walked into OB and asked for pain meds. I had been up all night, leaking amniotic fluid and having contractions. I was given pain meds and later high doses of Pitocin to move the labor along, which did not work. I ended up with a C-Section. Was I disappointed it went that way? I wasn't real crazy about all the pain from the Pitocin but I delivered a healthy baby girl.

As Stephanie neared the end of her pregnancy, she was asked about her birth plan. She had researched pain meds and epidurals. She thought both sounded like a great idea. She answered, "I want a healthy baby." She, too, leaked all night and had to go to the hospital due to low amniotic fluid. She was induced with Pitocin. As the labor progressed, she requested an epidural. The nurses said she needed to be hydrated first. They opened up the IV and the labor continued. They gave her an IV pain med which helped. Stephanie requested the epidural again but the anesthesiologist was in surgery; she would have to wait. The labor progressed. All of a sudden, she was dilated to eight. She requested the epidural, again. Too late. She requested more pain meds. Too late. Stephanie was dilated to ten and requested a C-section. "No indication for a C-section," the doctor said. Stephanie pushed four times and Amelia came into this world.

Stephanie had a birth plan. She wanted to have minimal pain during labor and delivery with the help of an epidural. Was she disappointed she didn't have an epidural? No, because her primary goal was to give birth to a healthy baby girl, and she did.

If you feel you need a birth plan, this is what I suggest: First, check your modesty at the door. There will be fluids and sometimes stool that come out of you during the course of labor and delivery. This is normal. People will be checking you vaginally on a regular basis. Second, have a supportive person or persons with you during labor and delivery. This is imperative. Labor and delivery are tough. It is going to hurt. If someone tells you it is going to be "a little uncomfortable," do not believe them. You need someone by your side to help you through labor. Third, decide if you want to deliver at home with a midwife or at the hospital with a midwife or an obstetrician. How do you feel about pain meds, or an epidural? You may need them. If you are in so much pain you cannot function, the pain med or epidural can help the labor progress. You have not failed if you use pain medication. Bottom line, your birth plan is to have a baby in whatever way is required for a safe delivery.

It would have been foolhardy of me to have devised a birth plan that stated I would not have a C-section. My baby was in distress. She needed to get out of me fast; so I had a C-section. The end goal was achieved: a healthy, beautiful baby girl.

Throw out the birth plan and go have your baby.

SUPPLEMENTS

Ginger Root can be helpful for reducing nausea. Other measures include eating something salty before getting out of bed (saltine crackers work great) and eating protein at each meal.

Suggested Dose
Ginger Root — 250 mg four times per day

Probiotics help maintain a healthy gastro-intestinal system, improve metabolism and the immune system. They also have a positive effect on the baby. See page 106.

Suggested Dose
Metagenics Ultra Bifidus DF — ½ tsp per day. This provides 15 billion CFU bifidobacterium

Vitamin D3, good for you and the baby. Low Vitamin D during pregnancy increases the risk of fetal hypocalcaemia (low calcium) which can cause low bone density in the baby, and slower than normal growth during the first year of life. See page 108 for health benefits for adults.

Suggested Dose
Orthomolecular Vitamin D3 1000 IU — two capsules per day

Omega-3 fatty acid—Docosahexaenoic Acid (DHA)—is important for the development of the fetus's brain, vision, and central nervous system. DHA can also decrease the risk for postpartum depression. The other Omega-3 fatty acid, EPA, is also important for overall health. See page 103 for more benefits from Omega-3 fatty acids.

Suggested Dose
Metagenics EPA-DHA 750 Natural Citrus Flavor— two capsules per day. This provides 750 mg EPA + 750 mg DHA.

Pre-natal Vitamin

Bach Rescue Remedy for reducing anxiety during labor. See page 96.

Suggested Dose
Four drops under your tongue, hold in your mouth as long as you can, then swallow. Repeat every 20 minutes as needed. (Also helpful for Dad.)

Postpartum Depression

The feminine principles of connection, care, concern and community must prevail. The postpartum period is an inherently regressive time, when a women needs to depend on others for care, food, and safety . . . and allow others to care for her so she is freed to care for her baby.

~Deborah Sichel MD and Jeanne Watson Driscoll MS, RN, CS
Women's Moods: What Every Woman Must Know about Hormones, the Brain and Emotional Health

Even though most women refuse to admit they are depressed after having a baby, the fact is postpartum depression is on the rise. The baby blues, a mild form of postpartum depression, is common. This may be caused by unrealistic expectations about being the perfect mother, which are amplified by the post-delivery hormonal swings and sleep deprivation. Potential health problems which can add to postpartum depression include hypothyroidism, hyperthyroidism, anemia, and low Vitamin D.

How can you tell if you are suffering from postpartum depression? Since giving birth to your child:

- Do you blame yourself whenever something goes wrong?

- Have you felt scared or panicky for no apparent reason?

- Have you been anxious or worried for no apparent reason?

If you answered yes to these questions, seek help. You may need treatment with an antidepressant and/or counseling.

The risk factors for postpartum depression include:
- History of depression or bipolar disorder
- Depression during pregnancy
- Premenstrual mood syndrome
- Poor social support
- Poor partner relations
- Lack of a close confidante

- Social isolation

- Stressful life events

Other contributing factors are a loss of identity, financial independence, work status, and freedom.

I remember when I first read the quote on page 75, I realized the feminine principles of connection, care, concern, and community are needed for the prevention and treatment of postpartum depression. In the days of old, we lived in community, with family nearby. Women were cared for so they could care for their babies. Today many women are far away from their families and feel isolated and alone. Most have more than one young child to care for and must return to work fulltime soon after the baby is born. No wonder postpartum depression is on the rise.

Countless women feel guilty if they are depressed after giving birth and do not seek help. They wonder why they are not in complete joy about the birth of their baby.

Look at the numbers. You are not alone.

11.7% – 20.4% of women get postpartum depression

26% – 85% of new mothers get the baby blues

These statistics clearly show it is normal to not feel ecstasy after the birth of a baby.

What should you do? As mentioned above, if you are not doing well, seek professional help. Do this for yourself, your baby, and those around you. Get your labs checked, begin medication, start counseling. Do something!

Remember the rule: *Seek other Moms* to help you let go of the unrealistic expectations of being the perfect mom. Do what you must to get more sleep and find time for you.

For me, a complicated pregnancy and a baby at the age twenty-nine was a shock. I had always worked or gone to school and was in the midst of a master's degree program when I became pregnant. I assumed I would continue my life as is, and have a baby. Was I surprised! The changes in my life, which started with the complications of pregnancy and then giving birth, were immense. I was no longer in control of my life.

After three months at home with Stephanie, I started the final course for my master's degree and took a quilting class. Did I feel guilty about leaving my baby with a sitter? Yes. However, you must remember the first rule of parenting: *If mama ain't happy, nobody's happy.* I knew in my heart I was not stay-at-home-mom material, and I was supported by friends in this. Back to school and quilting class I went, where I felt some modicum of control. This filled me up and I was able to be a better mom.

WAYS TO ALLEVIATE THE BABY BLUES

Seek social support. Join a mom's group, meet with friends, go to church, go back to work, take a class. Seek other women.

Take a nap. It is okay to rest. According to a study done at the University of California at Berkeley, naps make you smarter.

Make time for you. The change in your life that occurs when you go from being pregnant to being a mom is something no one can explain to you. I imagined I would be the same person, only I would now also be a mom. Wrong! Everything changes. I once read the baby blues/postpartum depression is a grief response from the changes which occur in a woman's life. I believe there is truth to this. Every day take 20 minutes for you and 10 minutes for your partner, plus go on regular dates.

Exercise and eat well. Sleep deprivation, hormonal fluctuations, and stress can change your brain chemistry, which can cause anxiety, worry, and depression. Exercise helps balance brain chemistry, decreases depression and anxiety, and blows off stress. Eating a low-carbohydrate diet can bring balance to brain chemistry. Take a good multivitamin and a B-complex (50 to 100 mg daily).

> There are two types of moms in this world: Those who desire to stay at home and those who desire to work outside the home. Determine which one you are and honor yourself for your choice. Honor all women in their choice.

IT TAKES A VILLAGE

I get by with a little help from my friends.
~ The Beatles

There were many amazing people who helped raise my daughter. Find your support: in your family, in your community, wherever you can. You will never be the perfect mom, spouse, friend, employee, or volunteer. Do the best you can. Then accept yourself in all your imperfections, as you accept others.

If you know a young mother, offer your support in any way you can. In our fast-paced society, many women miss out on the feminine principles—connection, care, concern, and community. For a large part of my life I have been blessed with community. There have been times when I was lost and alone, wondering which way was up. Over time I realized I needed help and went in search of community.

Some women don't know how to find community. I ask you to seek out these women. Offer kindness. Say, "It's tough raising a baby, isn't it? How are you doing?" Listen. Let them talk. I remember making a presentation to a mom's group. At the end I was answering a question and they all started to talk. I thought, they don't want to listen to me. They need to talk with each other, and so they did.

Eating a Healthy Diet

Childhood obesity is best tackled at home through improved parental involvement, increased physical exercise, better diet and restraint from eating.
~ Bob Filner

There are a lot of unhealthy, unhappy parents raising unhealthy, unhappy kids. How can you have healthy and happy children? You can do this by changing *your* eating habits and engaging in physical activity. This must be a family effort. If you tell your kids to eat healthy and to exercise while you sit on the couch eating junk, they will ignore what you say and do as you do. Remember the rule: ***Your child is watching you, and she will mimic what you do.*** It takes effort to eat healthy because there are so many temptations. There are a lot of conflicting messages on what is and is not healthy to eat. This can be very confusing. I can tell you what I do and what I teach in my practice. If you make these changes you will be amazed at how good you can feel.

> ***Childhood obesity is leading to an increase in acute and chronic medical conditions with a decrease in self-esteem and increase in depression.***
> ~ JM Wieting, *Cause and Effect in Childhood Obesity: Solutions for a National Epidemic*

The medical community has reported a drastic increase in chronic diseases starting at younger ages and even in children. High cholesterol, diabetes, heart disease, cancer, and Alzheimer's disease are on the rise. All have links to insulin resistance which is caused by eating too many carbohydrates.

We are also seeing more polycystic ovarian syndrome which is linked to insulin resistance and obesity. Polycystic ovarian syndrome is a metabolic disease that affects the hormones. It can cause irregular periods, infertility, uterine cancer, heart disease, and diabetes. The treatment of choice is through a proper diet.

Gastro esophageal reflux disease (GERD) is becoming common in children. Treating GERD with a medication, such as a proton pump inhibitor, leads to nutrient deficiency and long-term health consequences. We are already seeing health consequences in adults from the long-term use of the proton pump inhibitor. The concern for children is they will be on the medication for a much longer period of time than adults. This puts them at higher risk for long-term health consequences. The treatment of choice is dietary changes. In adults, supplementation with digestive enzymes and Betaine HCl can be helpful to reduce the symptoms of GERD.

Anxiety and depression are also being linked to diet. Men and women have told me about a feeling of rage that occurs sometimes after they eat sugar. This is caused by a rise and fall in blood sugar and all the hormonal chaos a body goes through to bring itself back into balance.

I wonder how much Attention Deficit Disorder (ADD), Attention Deficit Hyperactivity Disorder (ADHD), and oppositional disorders are related to diet. When I talk with parents who have children with these disorders, I learn many are eating diets full of sugar and refined carbohydrates.

Hypoglycemia reactions are also becoming more common. (My daughter and I experience hypoglycemia if we do not eat a protein breakfast before drinking coffee. We must eat protein at each meal to keep our blood sugar stable.) Hypoglycemia can be frightening. Your mind does not say, "Attention! Attention! Blood sugar is starting to fall, go eat something!" Instead, you feel horrible for no apparent reason. It takes thirty to sixty minutes to recover and then you may experience a feeling of weakness. During the time blood sugar is low and recovery is in progress, you can experience shakiness, panic, irritability, rage, fast heartbeat, irregular heartbeat, shortness of breath, and fuzzy thinking.

Food sensitivities are on the rise and can cause a whole host of health problems. The most common culprits of food sensitivities are wheat, milk, corn, cheese, coffee, eggs, chocolate, nuts, and peanuts. If you are not feeling well, stop eating one of these foods for twenty-one days. Then reintroduce a good amount of that food into your diet on a day you can be at home. No effect? Then you can confidently add this food back into your diet. However, if the food affects you in an adverse way, eliminate it from your diet permanently.

Gluten, found in wheat, rye, barley, and oats can cause gluten sensitivity and Celiac Disease. There has been a dramatic increase in Celiac Disease, an autoimmune disease. I also see a lot of gluten sensitivity in my patients, which causes them to not feel well. Removing gluten from your diet can have a dramatic effect on the health of you and your children.

TAKE CHARGE

Every small positive change we make in ourselves
repays us in confidence in the future.
~ Alice Walker

Following are suggestions to help you and your family move towards healthier eating. I know no one likes change. Carbohydrates taste good. I am a carbohydrate addict. What I have learned is I feel fabulous when I am off refined carbohydrates and I feel horrible when I eat them. I am still learning to make the choice day after day after day.

Take charge of your household. You are making these changes to benefit yourself and your children. This intervention is nothing more than a healthier diet and regular exercise. All family members must participate; this is a group effort. You must work together in the kitchen. Have a brainstorming session on healthier foods and eating habits everyone can partake in.

Start tomorrow. Remember the rule: *When training your child in new behavior, it may take up to a week of torture before she accepts and embraces it.* Keep calm and carry on. Persevere. Stand your ground when moving your family to healthier eating. Our children will die young unless there is a drastic change in what we feed them.

Make sure your children take at least two bites of every food on their plate before they can leave the table. If they turn up their noses and say "Ew! What's this?" tell them what it is. If they still refuse to eat it, send them away from the table. They will not starve from missing a meal and you can eat in peace.

MAKE IT A GAME

Gamification means taking an ordinary task (running, losing weight) and adding a game layer to it, like points, levels, badges. It isn't about making real life easier. It's about making real life more challenging, in ways that we want.

~Jane McGonigal, *Reality Is Broken: Why Games Make Us Better and How They Can Change the World*

85

Keep a chart denoting what activity and how long each person exercises on a daily basis. Post it on a wall or the refrigerator. Write down what everyone eats daily. Each family member can carry a notebook to monitor what he or she eats throughout the day. At the end of the week compare notes on the amount of exercise and how many deviations from healthy eating occurred for each individual.

Whoever has stayed with the healthiest program during the week is announced the winner. The winner gets a treat. She may get to eat on a special plate all week, pick a fun activity for the weekend, stay up past bedtime, or choose the music in the car. Make these healthy changes a fun game, with a little competition.

After the weekly winner has been announced, discuss what caused each family member to go astray from healthy eating and exercise. As a group, brainstorm what can be done to prevent it from happening the next time. When making life changes, it is important to remember the Five P's: Prior Proper Planning Prevents Problems.

THE TRUTH ABOUT CERTAIN FOODS

Artificial sweeteners should be avoided. They are neuro-excitatory chemicals which means they over-stimulate the brain. They are sweeter than sugar, thus more addictive. Research shows an association between the use of artificial sweeteners and obesity, diabetes, metabolic syndrome, and insulin resistance.

Bananas contain three types of sugar: glucose, sucrose, and fructose. People eat bananas because they want to increase their potassium intake. The sugar in the banana is worse for you than the benefit you get from potassium. If you need potassium, take an over-the-counter supplement or eat other high-potassium foods like green beans, Brussels sprouts, cantaloupe, honeydew melon, spinach, squash, Brazil nuts, and almonds. If you are on a high-protein diet you can lose potassium, which will manifest as muscle cramps. If you are on a water pill, your blood needs to be tested to check potassium levels. You may need to take a potassium medication replacement.

Broccoli. Can you hear your mom say, "Eat your broccoli"? Cruciferous vegetables—broccoli, cauliflower, Brussels sprouts, cabbage, and kale—have a healthy impact on genes and promote good health.

Carbohydrates, especially refined carbohydrates, should not make up the majority of your daily food intake. People tend to think pasta and bagels are better than donuts and chocolate. They are not. They are actually higher in carbohydrates.

- 1.5 ounces Pasta = 30.5 Gm carbohydrates
- 1.5 ounces Mini pretzels = 37.5 Gm carbohydrates
- 1.5 ounces M&Ms = 27 Gm carbohydrates
- Plain Bagel = 29 – 68 Gm carbohydrates
- Glazed Donut = 25 – 57 Gm carbohydrate
- Hershey's Milk Chocolate Bar = 26 Gm carbohydrates

Cheese, full fat, is good for you. It contains Vitamin K2 which reduces the risk of cancer and heart disease. Vitamin K2 also keeps bones and blood vessels healthy.

A recent study from France showed cheese and dairy products decreased the metabolic syndrome and diabetes over a nine year period. The mechanism of action is unknown.

Eggs are the perfect protein. Eat the yolk! Egg yolks contain choline, lutein, iron, and other vitamins and nutrients. Choline is converted to acytylcholine, a neurotransmitter, important for learning, memory, concentration, and perception. Lutein is important for eye health.

Fruit, in moderation, is good for you. You may eat one to two servings per day. One serving is one half cup. Fruit is loaded with sugar. Eat fruit for dessert or with a protein so you don't get the rise and fall of blood sugar.

Milk consumption is a risk factor for the developmnet of diabetes and a cause of acne. (It is not the chocolate!) Drinking milk with Vitamin D does not improve Vitamin D levels. The best source of Vitamin D is the sun or a supplement.

Nuts and peanuts in moderation are good for you. Moderation is 1 to 2 ounces (1/4 to 1/3 cup). Measure and then put the jar away in the cupboard!

Oatmeal, slow cooked, with nothing in it, reduces cholesterol by about 16 points. Flavored instant oatmeal, with all the sugar in it, will cause weight gain and increase blood sugar and cholesterol. I suggest avoiding oatmeal as it has very little protein in it.

Sugar alcohols are added to a product for sweetness without causing the same effect as sugar in the body. You will find sugar alcohols in protein bars, protein drinks, and several other products. In moderation, they are tolerable. In excess, they can cause gastrointestinal distress—severe bloating, gas, and abdominal pain.

Vegetables need to be a big part of your daily intake, excluding corn, peas, and potatoes. Potatoes have more sugar than sugar. You can eat sweet potatoes occasionally. This rule does not apply to fresh corn on the cob. During the month of August and early September, enjoy as much corn on the cob as possible with butter and salt!

Yogurt is full of sugar which feeds the bad bacteria and wipes out the good bacteria. Don't eat yogurt unless you make it yourself or buy plain yogurt and add one serving of fruit. I suggest eating cottage cheese or whole-milk ricotta cheese in place of yogurt. Both contain good amounts of protein and are low in carbohydrates.

HEALTHY EATING TIPS

★ If you want a sugar substitute use stevia or xylitol

★ Avoid eating low-fat products as they have simply replaced the fat with carbohydrates. People are actually gaining weight on these products. Eat full-fat foods.

★ Use butter, not margarine.

★ Buy food from the outer edge of the grocery store and skip the bakery.

★ When using protein shakes as a meal replacement, it is imperative to have mid-morning and mid-afternoon snacks. I drink a protein shake for breakfast (within an hour of waking and before caffeine). I have a protein bar mid-morning, a protein shake for lunch, and a cheese stick with nuts in mid-afternoon. Dinner is a vegetable and meat.

★ Be a timed eater. Eat at regular intervals throughout the day. If you don't, in the late afternoon or when you get home from work, you will open the refrigerator or cupboards and announce "let the eating begin."

Feeling Stuffer

Is eating a "feeling stuffer" for you? A feeling stuffer is an action or substance you use to avoid feeling. (Read *Invite Joy Into Your Life* by Mary B. Seger) Many foods are feeling stuffers. You will know a food is a feeling stuffer if you say "I deserve this" before indulging . . . and once you start to eat it, you cannot stop. For some people it is salty foods, for others it is sweets. Or, it could be both. My personal favorites are Peanut M&Ms and chocolate-covered peanuts.

If you want to be healthy you cannot eat these trigger foods because you have little or no control. I would like to say that in time you can eat your trigger foods in moderation. I have tested this theory many times and I have not been successful. If you are addicted to a type of food, the same as a smoker is to nicotine and an alcoholic is to drinking, a drug addict is to a drug, you cannot have that food.. Watch what you are teaching your children. Addictions are genetic and environmental.

★ Take the recommended supplements: Multivitamin, Omega-3s, Vitamin D, Probiotics, Fiber, and B Complex.

★ Drink water throughout the day.

★ Avoid drinking juice and sodas as they are full of sugar.

★ Taste buds can take up to six weeks to change and begin to appreciate healthy food. Keep calm and carry on!

BREAKFAST

Breakfast is the most important meal of the day. Eating breakfast is nonnegotiable for everyone in the family. Food should be eaten before drinking any caffeine. Drinking coffee or caffeinated tea on an empty stomach causes a rise and fall in blood sugar. When blood sugar goes up it over-stimulates the pancreas to produce insulin to lower the blood sugar. Over time, this can lead to hypoglycemic reactions and eventually diabetes. Hypoglycemia also affects the adrenal glands and causes a rise in cortisol. An increase in cortisol will increase the blood sugar and cause you to gain weight in your middle. As women age they become more sensitive to the rise and fall in cortisol, which can lead to weight gain without a change in diet. Sugar and white flour adversely affect your blood sugar and cortisol levels.

I suggest you eat a protein breakfast of eggs cooked to your preference, chicken, or a protein shake. You must eat the protein breakfast within one hour after waking up and before coffee. Feed your children a protein breakfast every day without exception. Remember the rule: *You are a parent, not your child's friend.*

Some breakfast suggestions:

★ Egg frittata

★ Hardboiled eggs

★ VRP Whey Protein Nutrition Shake—Chocolate or Vanilla (this product contains high-quality, undenatured whey protein). One scoop contains 20 grams of protein, 1 gram carbohydrate and is sweetened with stevia.

★ Baked chicken breast with cheese, salsa, or plain

★ Omelet

★ Ricotta pancakes

★ Fried, scrambled, or poached eggs

SNACKS

Provide healthy snacks after school. Children need fuel (food) every three to four hours. You do, too! Here are some easy snacks:

★ Apple with cheese, nuts, or peanut butter

★ Beef Jerky

★ Celery and peanut butter

★ Cheese stick

★ Cottage cheese

★ Deli roast beef, thinly sliced, with Schuler's Original Cheddar Cheese Spread

★ Fresh blueberries, raspberries, or strawberries with a cheese stick or nuts

- ★ Ham and cheese rolled around a dill pickle or a green onion

- ★ Ham and cream cheese

- ★ Hardboiled egg

- ★ Hummus with veggies

- ★ Nuts

- ★ Peanuts

- ★ Pepperoni with Swiss or mozzarella cheese

- ★ Fillo tarts with ham and cheese

- ★ Protein bar with at least fourteen grams of protein. My favorites are Zone, Cliff, Atkins, Metaplex and Balance. Read the labels to check for adequate protein amounts. Be aware of the effect of sugar alcohols on your body.

- ★ Sautéed nuts in butter with salt—it's better than popcorn!

- ★ Swiss cheese and almonds

- ★ Veggies and dip with cheese or nuts

LUNCH

- ★ Meat and cheese roll-up

- ★ Salad with protein and vegetables

- ★ Tuna fish, egg salad, or chicken salad on lettuce

- ★ VRP Whey Protein Nutrition Shake

DINNER

For a healthy dinner, serve meat and vegetables with one portion (half cup) of a starch. Teach your children to measure. Instead of using large dinner plates serve meals on salad plates. Allow space between each food item. Do not heap the plate full of food. Do not put the extra food on the table. If you want seconds, set the timer for 30 minutes. When it dings, assess whether you are truly hungry, if so eat more. If not, move away from the kitchen.

Some easy dinner suggestions:

★ Manwich in one pound of hamburger with cheese on top and a vegetable or salad on the side

★ Baked chicken from the grocery store with a fresh/frozen vegetable

★ Large salad with protein and vegetables

★ Taco Salad

★ Thanksgiving Dinner with turkey, squash, green bean casserole, and sweet potato pie. Use the leftover turkey for soup, salads, or turkey salad using the chicken salad recipe

★ Cut four boneless, skinless chicken breasts into small pieces. Stir-fry them in oil for four to five minutes. Remove from pan. Stir-fry three cups of chopped vegetables plus one small chopped onion in pan for four to five minutes. Add the chicken back into the pan, sprinkle with your favorite herbs, stir-fry for one to two minutes. Serve.

Supplements

The recommended pharmaceutical grade supplements
can be purchased at www.HealthyVitality.biz

BACH FLOWER REMEDIES

Bach Flower Remedies are homeopathic preparations made from the essence of plants. *Homeopathic* means they are diluted preparations, which means you are working with the energy of the plant. They are made in alcohol to keep the formulas stable; children's remedies contain no alcohol. There are no side effects, so you can't hurt yourself by taking them. I find these to be powerful emotional healers, especially in patients who are sensitive to traditional medications. To use Bach Flower Remedies, I suggest looking at the different remedies and picking three or four that apply to your current situation.

For descriptions of the Bach Flower Remedies visit www.bachflower.com. Also see suggested books under Recommended Reading.

Bach Rescue Remedy—I use Bach Rescue Remedy when I am stressed to the max. I also use it for sleep. It is a homeopathic remedy developed in the early 1900s by Dr. Bach. It contains Rock Rose for terror and panic; Impatiens for impatience and irritability; Clematis when not present mentally or spaced-out; Star of Bethlehem for trauma and shock; Cherry Plum for the verge of nervous breakdown or anger. (These are common feelings for most parents on any given day.) Bach Rescue Remedy is available in alcohol-based formula drops or spray.

Suggested Dose
Bach Rescue Remedy—four drops or one spray under tongue. Hold in mouth as long as you can, then swallow. May repeat every twenty minutes as needed.

Kids Rescue Remedy (Alcohol Free)

Suggested Dose
Kids Rescue Remedy—four drops under the tongue to be held in the mouth as long as possible before swallowing; or four drops added to a beverage. This can be repeated up to four times per day; pastilles are chewable and come in a handy tin.

Sleep Rescue Remedy and **Rescue Night Liquid Melts** (Alcohol Free) contain all of the above ingredients plus White Chestnut for a restless mind and help with repetitive thoughts. It could be used during the day when your mind will not stop.

Bach Emotional Eating Support Kit contains three remedies: Cherry Plum, to help you stay in control; Crab Apple, a cleansing remedy to help you feel better about yourself; Chestnut Bud, to help you change self-destructive patterns and allow you to choose healthier options.

Bach Kids Daydream Remedy (Alcohol Free) with Clematis is taken to treat indifference, boredom, or being spaced-out. It helps with grounding and focus.

Bach Kids Confidence Remedy (Alcohol Free) with Larch is given to children who doubt or don't believe in themselves, are hesitant and passive.

B-COMPLEX

Stress and some medications like birth control and Metformin, a diabetes medication, wipe out B Vitamins.

If this happens you can become fatigued and depressed. Many physicians treat this with an antidepressant. I suggest taking a B complex instead.

Folic acid, one of the B vitamins, promotes cervical health. The cervix is checked during a Pap test. When a woman has an abnormal pap smear, depending on the severity of the abnormality, we might prescribe prescription-strength folic acid for three to six months, then repeat the pap smear. To promote cervical health, take B complex which contains folic acid. B complex will turn your urine bright yellow. If it causes mild nausea, take it in the middle of a meal. If the nausea continues, stop taking the B complex.

Folic acid is important for the prevention of Spina bifida. It is recommended women take folic acid before becoming pregnant and during the pregnancy to promote a healthy neurological system in the baby.

Studies also show improved brain function and decreased dementia with supplementation of B12 and folic acid. If your lab work indicates you are low-normal, I suggest you take additional B12 and folic acid along with your B complex. The B vitamins are a family and work better when taken together. If you take a lot of one B vitamin it won't work as well and you won't get the benefit from the other B's, therefore a B complex is the best choice. Have lab work done in three months to see if this helps.

Some studies indicate that taking a B Complex with the herb Vitex can be helpful for the treatment of Premenstrual Syndrome (PMS). Vitex balances out estrogen and helps increase progesterone. It is a nutritive herb, so it is safe with minimal side effects. I have successfully treated PMS in my patients for years by suggesting Vitex. It can also help decrease menstrual cramping and flow, over time. When my daughter was a senior in high school, she started to take it. Life became more peaceful in our home.

I have also suggested Vitex for a basic treatment of infertility and have had great results.

Suggested Dose
PhysioLogics Vitex—two capsules per day

Orthomolecular Ortho B Complex—one to two capsules per day

Douglas Laboratories Sublingual-12 Plus—one per day. This provides extra B12 and folic acid in addition to the Ortho B Complex.

Warning: taking too many B vitamins can be toxic to the neurological system

CALCIUM

Calcium is important for healthy bones and teeth, blood vessels, muscle function, and nerve transmission. Vitamin D is needed for calcium absorption into the bone. Calcium absorption into the bone peaks in girls at age 12.5 and in boys at age 14. Bone mass is mostly achieved by age 18 and complete by age 28.

It is imperative to remember bone health begins in childhood, actually during pregnancy. Risk factors for osteoporosis (low bone mass) include age, sex, family history, smoking, drinking, estrogen deficiency (which can occur with anorexia and excessive physical exercise), small bone structure, sedentary lifestyle, low calcium and Vitamin D intake, depression, and various medications. Healthy bone promotion and osteoporosis prevention depend on a healthy diet, adequate calcium and Vitamin D intake, and exercise. This needs to begin during pregnancy.

For adults I recommend calcium citrate as it does not need to be taken with a meal in order to be absorbed into the body. It is also easily absorbed if you do not have good digestion. As we age, we produce less acid in our stomach and have decreased gastric enzyme production and function. This can lead to poor digestion and decreased absorption of nutrients.

Usually children can take calcium carbonate because they still have good digestion. The medical community is seeing diminished digestion in some children due to poor diet, which they are treating with medication. The medication, proton pump inhibitors (PPI), prevents the absorption of calcium, thus putting these children at risk for osteoporosis. We are already seeing this in adults along with other side effects secondary to the PPI medication and reduced nutrient absorption.

Most children and adults do not get enough calcium in their diets and need to take supplements.

The Food and Nutrition Board at the Institute of Medicine of the National Academies recommends these dosages of calcium:

> Children ages 4 to 8—1000 mg per day
> Children ages 9 to 18—1300 mg per day
> Adults ages 19 to 50—1000 mg per day

Calcium is in various foods, including:

> Plain yogurt, 8 ounces, 415 mg
> Swiss cheese, 1 ounce, 272.2 mg
> Mozzarella cheese, 1 ounce, 207 mg
> Cheddar cheese, 1 ounce, 204 mg
> Muenster cheese, 1 ounce, 203 mg

Suggested Dose
Adults—Douglas Laboratories Calcium Citrate—500 mg two times per day

Children—Vivactiv Calcium Chews—one chew with two meals per day. Do not give them more than the recommended amount as a side effect of calcium is constipation.

FIBER

Fiber is important for bowel health and normal bowel function. It may reduce the incidence of colon and rectal cancer. One study found that women who ate higher levels of soluble fiber had less occurrence of breast cancer; insoluble fiber had no association. Soluble fiber helps lower cholesterol and blood sugar. Insoluble fiber increases stool bulk and helps with constipation, irregular stools, and diarrhea. You can get some fiber in your foods, but most high-fiber foods are also high in carbohydrates. I suggest supplementing with a product that contains soluble and insoluble fiber.

The American Heart Association makes the following recommendations for fiber:

> Children ages 1 to 3—19 gm per day
> Children ages 4 to 8—25 gm per day

Females ages 9 to 18—26 gm per day
Males ages 9 to 13—31 gm per day
Males ages 14 to 18—38 gm per day
Adults—25 to 30 gm per day

Suggested Dose
Orthomolecular Fiber Plus—one to three capsules per
day with a minimum of one 8-ounce glass of water with
each capsule. This provides almost 6.5 Gm of soluble and
insoluble fiber in one capsule.

Children—Orthomolecular Fiber Plus—one to three
capsules per day with a minimum of one 8-ounce glass of
water per capsule.

FLAXSEED OIL

Flaxseed oil is an Omega-3 Fatty Acid. However, it is minimally converted to EPA and DHA, which are the beneficial Omega-3 fatty acids. Ground flaxseed is a fiber and an excellent treatment for constipation. It also has an estrogenic effect. Studies show a reduction in hot flashes and breast cancer. I recommend you grind it daily or, at the most, two to three days in advance, and store it in the refrigerator. Flaxseed goes rancid fairly quickly, so I am not crazy about the pre-ground meal. Flaxseed can be ground in a coffee grinder or an actual flaxseed grinder. Mix it in your protein shake or water, sprinkle it on a salad or cottage cheese. After you have eaten flaxseed, give yourself a big smile in the mirror to check for seeds in your teeth! An appropriate dose starts with one teaspoon per day, gradually increased to 1/4 cup per day. If you increase the dose too quickly, the side effect is bowel distress.

Flaxseed must be ground to have an effect on the body. Unground flaxseed has no effect, it goes straight through.

MULTIVITAMIN

Adults and children need a good multivitamin because the foods we eat do not provide sufficient nutrients. The fresh vegetables and fruit I get from my brother's organic garden and the farmer's market in no way compare nutritionally to the vegetables and fruit I get at the grocery store, which is where most of us shop.

Suggested Dose
Adults—Orthomolecular Alpha Base capsules without iron—four capsules per day. If you are in poor health, take four capsules two times per day. Do not take a multivitamin with iron unless you have a blood test to determine you are low in iron.

Children—Orthomolecular SuperNutes—two chewable capsules per day.

OMEGA-3 FATTY ACIDS

Omega-3 fatty acids have an anti-inflammatory effect and most, if not all, diseases have an inflammatory component. There are numerous studies showing the benefits of Omega-3 fatty acids in a variety of healthy aspects and disease states including heart health, osteoarthritis, rheumatoid arthritis, lupus, fibromyalgia, cancer prevention, depression, ADD, ADHD and healthy skin. I suggest everyone take Omega-3 fatty acids for good health and disease prevention. EPA and DHA are the Omega-3 fatty acids that have an anti-inflammatory effect in our bodies. DHA is most important for children and is now added to infant formula. When shopping for an Omega-3 fatty acid product, look for the amount of EPA and DHA. The suggested dose for adults is 1,000 to 2,000 milligrams of EPA + DHA per day, with doses up to 4,000 milligrams and higher per day for specific diseases. For adults you want a higher ratio of EPA:DHA. DHA is important during pregnancy to promote eye and brain development in the fetus. Some studies have shown DHA may prevent postpartum depression. EPA is important for overall health. Children may take a higher ratio of DHA:EPA because it continues to be important for eye and brain development. There have been numerous studies done using DHA to help treat ADD and ADHD. The results are mixed. I think it is worth a try. **Do not stop your child's medications without consulting with your healthcare provider.**

Before purchasing an Omega-3 product read the supplement facts label. Many times it will say on the front of the bottle: Fish Oil/Omega-3 1000 mg. However, when you look at the supplement facts there may only be 180 mg EPA and 120 mg DHA. My new favorite labeling is EPA + DHA + other Omega-3 fatty acids 480 mg. The "other Omega-3 fatty acids" have little to no affect in your body and you have no idea how much EPA and DHA you are getting.

Suggested Dose
Adults—Metagenics EPA-DHA 750 Natural Citrus Flavor —two capsules per day. This provides 750 mg EPA + 750 mg DHA . This is an adequate amount for pregnant women.

Infants—Breastfeeding moms need a minimum of 300 mg DHA in order to pass it on to their baby. Infant formula now contains DHA.

Children—Orthomega Pearls contain DHA 185 mg + EPA 105 mg per four gel capsules. To calculate the correct dose for your child, use one of the following formulas listed below.

Young's Rule

$$\frac{\text{Adult Dose x Child's Age}}{\text{Childs' Age} + 12}$$

Example for a 4-year-old child

$$\frac{1000 \text{ mg Omega-3 fatty acid x 4}}{4 + 12} = \frac{4000}{16} = 250 \text{ mg Omega-3 fatty acid}$$

Clark's Rule

$$\frac{\text{Weight of child in pounds x Adult Dose}}{150}$$

Example for a 30-pound child

$$\frac{30 \text{ pounds x 1000 mg of Omega-3 Fatty Acid}}{150} = \frac{30{,}000}{150} = 200 \text{ mg DHA/EPA}$$

Buyer Beware! There are foods advertised as containing Omega-3 fatty acids. A yogurt advertised for children contains 16 mg of DHA, a miniscule amount. An orange juice contains 50 mg of EPA and DHA combined, in eight ounces. Both products contain a lot of sugar and minimal Omega-3s.

PROBIOTICS

Probiotics are beneficial bacteria that promote gastro-intestinal health. The bacteria that have been studied the most are lactobacillus, bifidobacterium, and saccharomyces which is a beneficial yeast probiotic. I recommend a product that contains all three. For pregnant women, breastfeeding moms, infants, and children under two, I recommend bifidobacterium, the most prevalent bacteria in a baby's bowel up to age two.

Probiotics are good for your metabolism, nutrition, and the immune system. They also promote good bowel function. They must be taken on a regular basis because our environment does not otherwise support a healthy gut. Probiotics live in the gut for about thirteen days, therefore daily supplementation is necessary.

In *Natural Medicine, Optimal Wellness*, Dr. Alan Gaby states ". . . probiotics may be useful for preventing and/or treating the following conditions: antibiotic-induced diarrhea, colic, constipation, Crohn's disease, diverticular disease, flatulence, irritable bowel syndrome, ulcerative colitis, candidiasis, Clostridium difficile, urinary tract infection and vaginitis. A healthy gut needs a good probiotic, mixed fiber, and a look at food sensitivities."

In Probiotics in Children, *Pediatric Clinics of North America 54* (2007), Doctors Kligler, Hanaway, and Cohrssen suggest use of probiotics in children for prevention of antibiotic associated diarrhea, treatment of acute diarrhea, prevention of community acquired diarrhea, irritable bowel syndrome, constipation, infantile colic, and atopic dermatitis (prevention and treatment).

The American Academy of Pediatrics published a clinical report in *Pediatrics* (November 29, 2010) regarding Probiotics:

> *More research is needed but encouraging preliminary results regarding the use of probiotics and prebiotics in children find they may be helpful for H pylori, gastritis, irritable bowel syndrome, chronic ulcerative colitis, colic, common infections and atopy* (a genetic tendency to develop classic allergic disease—atopic dermatitis, allergic rhinitis, asthma). *They may also be helpful for antibiotic associated diarrhea.* (Take probiotic two hours apart from antibiotic). *They should not be administered to children with chronic or serious disease, immunocompromised, chronically debilitated or with indwelling medical devices.*

Suggested Dose

Colic
5–10 billion CFU per day

Antibiotic
20–25 billion CFU per day, two hours apart from antibiotic for six weeks

Irritable bowel syndrome
25–100 billion CFU, two times per day for six to eight weeks. Start at low dose and gradually increase. Maintenance Dose—20–25 billion CFU per day

Daily Maintenance
Adults—10–20 billion CFU
Children—5–10 billion CFU

*Adults—Orthomolecular Orthobiotic—one capsule per day.
This provides 20 billion CFU combined Lactobacillus and
Bifidobacterium + 2 billion CFU Saccharomyces.*

*Children over age two—Orthomolecular Flora Boost—one
to two scoops per day, mix in applesauce. This provides 5
billion CFU combined Lactobacillus and Bifidobacterium
and 1 billion CFU Saccharomyces in one scoop.*

*Children age two and under—Metagenics Ultra Bifidus
DF 1/8 to 1/4 teaspoon per day, mix in formula or
applesauce. This provides 7.5 billion CFU Bifidobacterium
in 1/4 teaspoon.*

*Pregnant women and breastfeeding moms—Metagenics
Ultra Bifidus DF 1/2 teaspoon per day. This provides 15
billion CFU Bifidobacterium.*

**Buyer Beware! Most yogurts with probiotics do
not contain therapeutic doses of probiotic. They
also contain a lot of sugar which feeds the bad
bacteria and wipes out the good bacteria**

VITAMIN D

Vitamin D receptors are in every cell in the human
body. Some of the effects of adequate Vitamin D levels
are healthy bones, increased immune system, decreased
dementia and depression, decreased risk of colon cancer,
breast cancer, and autoimmune diseases. Do not drink
milk for Vitamin D. Your best source of Vitamin D is the
sun or a supplement.

Your body makes Vitamin D when skin is exposed to the sun. Sunscreen as low as an SPF 8 blocks all production of Vitamin D. In my practice, I check blood work using the lab test 25 (OH) Vitamin D. The blood level of Vitamin D3 should be in the range of 60 to 100. In Northern Michigan, most people have Vitamin D levels in the 20s or below. In these cases, I have patients supplement with high doses of Vitamin D for three months to get their blood levels up, and then decrease the amount to a lower, maintenance dose. High doses of Vitamin D should not be taken unless blood work indicates it is needed. Vitamin D3 is the active vitamin D in the body. There are Vitamin D2 over-the-counter supplements and prescription medication. Studies show it is better to use Vitamin D3.

Suggested Dose
Adults—Orthomolecular Vitamin D3 1000 IU—2000 IU in the winter, 1000 IU in the summer if you are getting exposure to the sun without sunscreen. The Institute of Medicine recommended dietary allowance 600 IU, upper level intake 4,000 IU;

Pregnant Moms—Orthomolecular Vitamin D3 1000 IU—2000 IU per day or check blood work to determine if a higher dose is required. The Institute of Medicine recommended dietary allowance 600 IU, upper level intake 4,000 IU;

Breastfeeding Moms—Orthomolecular Vitamin D3 1000 IU—2000 IU per day or check blood work to determine if higher dose is needed. The Vitamin D content of breast milk is related to mom's Vitamin D status. Studies have shown high doses of Vitamin D supplements are needed to transfer Vitamin D in breast milk to ensure the infant receives an adequate amount of Vitamin D. Studies have not been done to determine what this dose should be, therefore breastfed infants should be supplemented with Vitamin D. The Institute of Medicine recommended dietary allowance 600 IU, upper level intake 4,000 IU;

Breastfed Infants, Children, Adolescents—Biotics Research Bio-D-Mulsion. This provides 400 IU Vitamin D3 per drop. The Institute of Medicine's recent recommendations: Infants 0-6 months no recommended dietary allowance, upper level intake 1000 IU; Infants 6-12 months no recommended dietary allowance, upper level intake 1,500 IU; 1-3 years old recommended dietary allowance 600 IU, upper level intake 2,500; 4-8 years old recommended dietary allowance 600 IU, upper level intake 3,000 IU; 9-18 years old recommended dietary allowance 600 IU, upper level intake 4,000 IU

Lavender Essential Oil

*Aromatherapy—the controlled use of essential oils
to maintain and promote physical, psychological,
and spiritual well-being.*

~ Gabriel Mojay

The first time I used lavender was during the Arsenic Hour. We were in the midst of bath time. Stephanie was crying and I was beside myself. Then I remembered lavender. I grabbed the bottle of lavender essential oil and put two drops in the tub. The phone rang. I went to answer the phone and all of a sudden there was complete silence. I ran back to the bathroom thinking Stephanie had drowned. There sat my sweet girl, peacefully inhaling the scent of lavender. Ahhhh. We used lavender every night thereafter.

Essential oils are concentrated, pure herbal oils used to treat physical and emotional ailments through inhalation or massage. All oils, except lavender, must be mixed with carrier oil when applied to the skin. Lavender can be applied neat, which means it is safe to use directly on the skin. Lavender is used to calm and soothe nerves. For tension headaches, apply one drop of lavender essential oil to each temple, sit down, take some deep breaths, and relax. For stress reduction, a couple drops in the bathwater will soothe jangled nerves.

One mom told me she carries a bottle of lavender essential oil in her purse when traveling with her kids. When the kids start to get noisy, she pulls out the bottle of lavender, takes a sniff and passes it around for all of her children to inhale. Peace reigns.

I have also put a drop of lavender under my nose when I am exposed to malodorous smells; all I smell is lavender. Life is good.

Recipes

This section contains some of the recipes I have collected and used over the years. You only need eight to ten recipes to offer a good variety.

BREAKFAST

Cottage Cheese and Berry Mix

In a bowl or tall glass, layer

½ cup cottage cheese

¼ cup fresh berries

1 tablespoon sunflower seeds

Egg Frittata

10 to 12 large eggs

½ cup half and half or ½ cup salsa

Beat ingredients together. Pour into sprayed pie plate. Suggested items to sprinkle into the frittata: grated cheese (mix in and sprinkle some on the top), diced ham, cooked sausage or bacon, sautéed vegetables such as onions, green/red/orange pepper, tomato, asparagus, mushrooms. Bake at 350 degrees for 50 minutes, in a sprayed pie plate.

Ricotta Cheese Pancakes

9 eggs

3 cups whole milk ricotta cheese

2 teaspoons vanilla extract

1½ teaspoons cinnamon

Whisk all ingredients together; grill as pancakes. Before serving top with fruit spread, lemon curd, butter, peanut butter, or strawberries and Reddi-wip—a decadent way to start the day!

LUNCH

Chicken Salad

6 chicken breasts, baked

1 cup of celery, diced

1 cup of mayonnaise

Let the chicken breasts cool and then chop into small pieces. Add the celery and mayonnaise. Stir together. Place on a bed of lettuce before serving.

Variations: Add basil, rosemary, oregano, thyme, sage, lemon pepper, olives, artichoke hearts, curry with raisins, dried cherries, dried cranberries, raisins, walnuts, pecans, and/or slivered almonds.

My favorite combos for chicken salad are:

Basil, celery, and slivered almonds

Apple, celery, and walnuts

Kalamata olives, artichoke hearts, and celery

Dried cherries, celery, and slivered almonds

Curry, raisins, and celery

Tuna Salad

2 small cans of tuna, drained

Mayonnaise, to taste

Mix together. Place on a bed of lettuce or eat plain. Add celery and onion if desired.

Egg Salad

Use the egg yolks! Add chopped celery and onion if desired. Serve on a bed of lettuce or eat plain.

DINNER

Green Salad

In the summer, I love to make a large salad for dinner and in the winter a side salad is a great addition to most meals. Because I find serving only greens to be amazingly boring, I add whatever I can find in the fridge. Different flavors and textures bring great joy to my taste buds. Note: use full-fat salad dressing because low-fat dressings have more carbohydrates.

Pick one or more items from each of the six categories:

Meat—chicken, turkey, ham, beef, tuna, salmon

Boiled eggs

Cheese, any type—my favorite is goat cheese, slightly warmed in the microwave

Fruit—strawberries, blueberries, raspberries, dried cherries, dried cranberries, apple, pear

Vegetables—green/red/ orange peppers, celery, tomato, broccoli, cauliflower, onion, avocado, carrot, radish, green beans, mushrooms

Nuts—walnuts, pecans, peanuts, cashews, and my favorite pine nuts

Some tasty combos:
Greens, chicken, goat cheese, pine nuts, celery, red pepper, dried cherries

Greens, chicken, parmesan cheese, walnuts, celery, red pepper, carrots, dried cherries

Greens, ham, turkey, boiled egg, broccoli, cauliflower, apple, walnuts

Greens, roast beef, cheddar, strawberries, celery, onion, broccoli, cauliflower, walnuts

Greens, chicken, cheddar cheese, avocado, celery, red pepper, pecans, dried cherries

Bill Baughman's BBQ Pork Steak

2 pork steaks

Barbeque sauce, your choice

Onion, sliced

Place pork steaks in baking pan, top with BBQ sauce and chopped onion. Bake at 350 degrees for 30 minutes; flip meat, top with more BBQ sauce. Bake 30 more minutes.

Lasagna

Spaghetti Squash

1 pound ground beef

1 onion, chopped

16 ounces spaghetti sauce

15-ounce container cottage cheese

1 egg

2 to 4 cups mozzarella cheese, shredded

Bake spaghetti squash for one hour; remove from shell and sauté in coconut oil. Brown the ground beef with the onion. Add spaghetti sauce and sautéed spaghetti squash to cooked ground beef. In a separate bowl, mix the cottage cheese with the egg.

Layer in a 13 x 9-inch pan, as follows:
Meat mixture
Cottage cheese mixture
Mozzarella cheese
Meat mixture
Mozzarella cheese

Refrigerate for 24 hours. Bake covered for one hour at 350 degrees. Serve with salad.

Chicken and Squash Stew

One roasted chicken from the grocery store. Remove skin and meat from bones; dice.

Sauté together:

4 cups of squash, any variety, peeled and diced

2 cups green beans, fresh or frozen

2 stalks celery, chopped

1 orange or red pepper, seeded and diced

1 onion, diced

Add chicken and veggies to a large pot with 8 cups of chicken broth. Simmer all day, stirring occasionally.

Pizza Pie

1 pound ground beef or 5 chicken breasts

Onion, diced

14 ounces pizza sauce

Mozzarella cheese, shredded

Your favorite pizza toppings

Brown ground beef with one onion or bake 5 chicken breasts and dice. Mix with 14 ounces of pizza sauce. Place in baking dish; top with your favorite pizza toppings and cheese. Bake at 350 degrees for one hour.

Beef Soup

Roast a three-pound boneless roast beef in a covered baking pan at 350 degrees for one and one half hours. Before roasting top with Montreal Steak Seasoning. Dice when cooled and place in large pot with seven cups of beef broth.

Sauté:

1 onion, diced

1 red pepper, seeded and diced

2 stalks of celery, chopped

8 ounces of mushrooms, sliced

1 small sweet potato, diced

Add sautéed veggies to the large pot. Simmer for at least two to three hours or all day, stirring occasionally. 30 minutes before serving, add 1 teaspoon each of basil and thyme.

Ground Beef, Swiss, and Mushroom Casserole

One pound ground beef

8-oz package mushrooms, sliced

Onion, diced

3 eggs, beaten slightly

3 cups Swiss cheese

Brown ground beef, sliced mushrooms, and diced onion. Place in 9 x 9 baking dish. Mix three eggs with two cups of the Swiss cheese; pour over meat mixture and top with remaining one cup shredded cheese. Bake at 350 degrees for one hour.

Taco Casserole

One pound ground beef

One medium onion, diced

One green pepper, seeded and diced

Taco Seasoning, your choice

16-oz can black beans, drained and rinsed

Tomato, chopped

Lettuce

Sour cream

Cheese, shredded

Salsa

Brown ground beef with onion and green pepper. Add one package of taco seasoning with recommended amount of water. Mix in rinsed black beans. Place mixture in a baking dish and cover with a layer of chopped tomatoes. Top with shredded cheese. Bake at 350 degrees for one hour. Serve with sour cream, salsa, and chopped lettuce

Grandma Gail's Chicken Broccoli Casserole

3 cups cooked chicken breasts, diced

2 small packages frozen broccoli (cooked and drained)

½ cup mayonnaise

1 can cream of chicken soup

1 teaspoon lemon juice

½ teaspoon curry powder

½ cup cheese, grated

Layer chicken and broccoli; mix rest of ingredients and pour over top of chicken and broccoli; top with ½ cup grated cheese. Bake at 350 degrees for one hour.

VEGETABLES

Green Bean Casserole – Mix 2 cans green beans with one can cream of mushroom soup, spoon into baking dish. Top with French fried onions. Bake at 350 degrees for 45 minutes.

Sweet Potato Pie – 3 large sweet potatoes, peeled and cut into medium-sized pieces. Boil until tender. Mash. Mix in 4 tablespoons butter, and 1 teaspoon each of vanilla extract, cinnamon, and nutmeg. Place in baking dish and top with pecan pieces. Bake at 350 degrees for one hour.

Spaghetti squash with butter and parmesan cheese

Green beans and onion sautéed with slivered almonds and lemon pepper

Broccoli and/or **cauliflower**, butter, shredded cheddar cheese

Vegetable Sauté – onions, mushrooms, orange pepper, and zucchini sautéed in coconut oil

Brussels sprouts or **asparagus** – steamed and served with butter

Squash – baked and served with butter

SNACKS

Bill Baughman's Sautéed Nuts

1 cup nuts (pecans or walnuts)

2 tablespoons of butter

Sauté nuts in melted butter in a large frying pan over medium heat; stirring frequently. Place in bowl, salt to taste. Enjoy. This is better than popcorn!

Fillo Tarts

Mini Fillo Shells (in frozen section)

Deli Ham, chopped

Colby Jack cheese, small slices

Honey Mustard

Place shells on baking sheet. Fill with ham, place a dollop of honey mustard on top of the ham and top with a slice or chunk of cheese. Bake at 350 degrees for five minutes.

Grandma Gail's Veggie Dip

1 cup mayonnaise

1 cup sour cream

1 teaspoon seasoned salt

2 drops Tabasco sauce

1½ teaspoons Worcestershire sauce

1 teaspoon dill weed

1 tablespoon minced onion

1 teaspoon seasoned salt

1 tablespoon parsley flakes

Mix together; pour in glass container. Chill at least 8 hours before serving.

DESSERTS

Sometimes you need something sweet. If you eat dessert immediately after a meal you won't get a rise and fall of blood sugar, or the hormonal chaos that goes with it. The protein and fat from your meal will maintain your blood sugar. You also can't eat as much. Use small bowls or plates.

Fruit is a great dessert. It offers the sweet taste along with vitamins and antioxidants. Remember fruit is full of sugar, measure ½ cup into a small bowl and enjoy!

The following recipes have been in my family for many years. Dessert is a tradition in my family. This started in my childhood as I come from a long line of bakers. The Christmas dessert spread at my Grandma's was a delight to behold! We carry on this tradition with yummy birthday cakes and Christmas cookies and bread. Find your old family recipes and share them with your children on holidays or other special occasions. Breaking bread or eating cake is a wonderful family tradition to be enjoyed in moderation. Remember the rule: *Start traditions.*

Fresh Strawberries & Reddi-wip

Remove hulls and wash strawberries. Shake dry and cut in half. Place strawberries in a bowl and put on the table with the Reddi-wip. Pick up a strawberry and spray Reddi-wip on it. The goal is to see how high you can get the Reddi-wip and still get the strawberry in your mouth.

Fruit Salad

Select four to five different fruits, chop into bite-sized pieces. Squirt a small amount of lemon juice over the fruit and stir. Serve in small bowl and enjoy!

Peanut Butter Blossoms

½ cup peanut butter

½ cup sugar

½ cup butter, softened

½ cup brown sugar

1 egg

1 teaspoon vanilla extract

1 teaspoon baking soda

½ teaspoon salt

1¾ cups flour

1 package chocolate kisses or chocolate stars

Cream together the first four ingredients; add egg and vanilla. Mix well. In a separate bowl, combine flour, salt and soda. Add dry mixture to other ingredients. Chill dough for at least two hours. Shape into one-inch balls and roll in granulated sugar. Bake at 375 degrees for 6 to 8 minutes. Press in candy kisses and bake an additional 2 to 5 minutes.

Texas Sheet Cake ~ Grandma Gail

In a saucepan, slowly bring to a boil:

1 cup butter (two sticks)
4 tablespoons cocoa powder
1 cup water

In a bowl, mix together:

2 cups flour
2 cups sugar
½ teaspoon salt

Pour butter mixture into bowl of dry ingredients. Mix well; then add:

2 eggs
½ cup sour cream
1 teaspoon baking soda

Mix well; then pour into a greased and floured 18 x 13 x 1 inch baking pan. Bake for 20 to 22 minutes (no longer) at 375 degrees. Frost the cake as soon as it comes out of the oven.

Frosting

In a saucepan, bring to a boil:

½ cup butter (one stick)
4 tablespoons cocoa powder
6 tablespoons milk

Add 1 pound powdered sugar. Mix well.

Add 1 teaspoon vanilla extract
1 cup chopped nuts (optional)

Start making the frosting five to ten minutes before the cake is ready to remove from the oven.

Apple or Strawberry Bread

   2 cups sugar

   3 cups flour

   1½ teaspoons baking soda

   1 teaspoon cinnamon

   1 teaspoon nutmeg

   3 cups chopped peeled apples or 3 cups chopped
   fresh strawberries

   1 cup chopped nuts (optional)

   3 eggs

   1¼ cups vegetable oil

   2 teaspoons vanilla extract

Combine ingredients. Spoon batter into two well-greased and floured bread pans. Bake one hour at 350 degrees. Check with toothpick to make sure it is done; may require 75 minutes to bake. Cool and store in refrigerator.

Pistachio Pudding ~ Grandma Rose

20-ounce can crushed pineapple, with juice

3-ounce box instant Pistachio pudding

1 cup mini-marshmallows

1 cup whipped topping

Maraschino cherries

Mix, chill, and enjoy!

Pistachio Bread ~ Aunt Joan

1 package yellow cake mix

3-ounce box instant Pistachio pudding

4 eggs

½ cup vegetable oil

¼ cup water

½ cup sour cream

Cinnamon/sugar/chopped nuts mixture

Mix ingredients well. Grease two bread pans. Make a mixture of cinnamon, sugar, and chopped nuts to taste. In bread pans alternate batter and cinnamon-sugar-nut mix in layers, ending with cinnamon mix on top. Bake at 350 degrees until done (one hour or less).

Carrot Cake

1½ cups vegetable oil

4 eggs

2 cups sugar

2 cups flour

2 teaspoons baking powder

2 teaspoons baking soda

1½ teaspoons salt

1 teaspoon cinnamon

3 cups grated carrots

Mix above ingredients. Pour into greased and floured 13 x 9-inch pan. Bake at 350 degrees for 45 minutes or until done.

Cream Cheese Frosting

1 8-ounce package cream cheese

½ cup butter (one stick)

1 pound confectioner's sugar

1 teaspoon vanilla extract

Mix ingredients; frost cooled cake.

Chocolate Cake with Peanut Butter Frosting

Chocolate Cake Mix

Follow directions. Bake in two round cake pans.

Peanut Butter Frosting

2 cups powdered sugar

1 cup butter, softened

2 cups smooth peanut butter

½ cup half and half

6 ounces cream cheese

1 teaspoon vanilla extract

Cream all ingredients except powdered sugar. Then add powdered sugar. Beat until smooth. Frost cooled chocolate cake.

Angel Food Cake with Cherries ~ Grandma Gail

Angel Food Cake

Cool Whip – one container

Cherry Pie Filling – one can

Place angel food cake on a serving plate, frost with Cool Whip. Spoon cherry pie filling over the top of the cake.

Resources

WEBSITES
www.MarySeger.com
www.RadiantRecovery.com
www.UVAdvantage.org
www.VitaminDCouncil.org

E-NEWSLETTER
Something to Contemplate – sign up at
    www.MarySeger.com

PHARMACEUTICAL GRADE SUPPLEMENTS
www.HealthyVitality.biz

BOOKS
Bach E. & Wheeler F.J. *The Bach Flower Remedies* (three books in one volume). Keats Publishing Inc., 1979.

Cruise J. *The Belly Fat Cure.* Hay House Inc., 2009.

DesMaisons K. *Little Sugar Addicts.* Three Rivers Press, 2004.

Gladwell M. *Blink: The Power of Thinking Without Thinking.* Little, Brown, and Company, 2005.

Howard J. *The Bach Flower Remedies: Step by Step.* C W Daniel Company Limited, 1990.

Northrup C. *Mother-Daughter Wisdom: Creating a Legacy of Physical and Emotional Health.* Bantam Books, 2005.

Northrup C. *Women's Bodies, Women's Wisdom: Creating Physical and Emotional Health and Healing.* Bantam Books, 1995.

Scheffer M. *Bach Flower Therapy: Theory and Practice.* Healing Arts Press, 1988.

Seger Mary B. *Invite Joy into Your Life: Steps for Women Who Want to Rediscover the Simple Pleasures of Living.* Sophia Rose Press, 2007.

Strand R. *Healthy for Life: Developing Healthy Lifestyles That Have a Side Effect of Permanent Fat Loss.* Real Life Press, 2005.

References

DIET

Benson LJ, Baer HJ, Kaelber DC. Screening for obesity-related complications among obese children and adolescents: 1999-2008. *Obesity* (9 December 2010)

Borushek A. *The Calorie King Calorie Fat and Carbohydrate Counter.* 2009. Costa Mesa CA: Family Health Publications.

Bügel S. Vitamin K and bone health in adult humans. *Vita Horm.* 2008;78:393-416.

Can AS, Uysal C., Palaoglu KE. Short term effects of a low-carbohydrate diet in overweight and obese subjects with low HDL-C levels. *BMC Endocr Disord.* 2010; 10: 18.

Davis NJ, Tomuta N, Schechter C, Isasi CR, Segal-Isaacson CJ, Stein D, Joel Zonszein, MD,[2] and Judith Wylie-Rosett, EDD, RD. Comparative Study of the Effects of a 1-Year Dietary Intervention of a Low-Carbohydrate Diet Versus a Low-Fat Diet on Weight and Glycemic Control in Type 2 Diabetes. *Diabetes Care.* 2009 July; 32(7): 1147–1152

Fodor D, Albu A, Poanta L, Porojan M. Vitamin K and vascular calcifications. *Acta Physiol Hung.* 2010 Sep;97(3):256-66.

Foster GD, Wyatt HR, Hill JO, PhD, Makris AP, Rosenbaum DL, Brill C, Stein RI, B. Mohammed S, Miller B, Rader DJ, Zemel B, Wadden TA, Tenhave

T, Newcomb CW, Klein S. Weight and Metabolic Outcomes After 2 Years on a Low-Carbohydrate Versus Low-Fat Diet A Randomized Trial *Ann Intern* Med. 2010 August 3; 153(3): 147–157.

Galletly C, Moran L, Noakes M, Clifton P, Tomlinson L, Norman R. Psychological benefits of a high-protein, low-carbohydrate diet in obese women with polycystic ovary syndrome--a pilot study. *Appetite.* 2007 Nov;49(3):590-3. Epub 2007 Apr 4.

Gast GC, de Roos NM, Sluijs I, Bots ML, Beulens JW, Geleijnse JM, Witteman JC, Grobbee DE, Peeters PH, van der Schouw YT. A high menaquinone intake reduces the incidence of coronary heart disease. *Nutr Metab Cardiovasc Dis.* 2009 Sep;19(7):504-10. Epub 2009 Jan 28.

Green PHR. Celiac Disease – *A hidden epidemic.* 2010. New York NY: William Morrow.

Guh DP, Zhang W, Bansback N, Amarsi Z, Birmingham CL, Anis AH. The incidence of co-morbidities related to obesity and overweight: a systematic review and meta-analysis. *BMC Public Health.* 2009 Mar 25;9:88.

Haimoto H, Sasakabe T, Wakai K, Umegaki H. Effects of a low-carbohydrate diet on glycemic control in outpatients with severe type 2 diabetes *Nutr Metab* (Lond). 2009; 6: 21. Published online 2009 May 6.

Halton TL, Liu S, Manson JE, Hu FB Low-carbohydrate-diet score and risk of type 2 diabetes in women. *Am J Clin Nutr.* 2008 February; 87(2): 339–346.

Nimptsch K, Rohrmann S, Kaaks R, Linseisen J. Dietary vitamin K intake in relation to cancer incidence and mortality: results from the Heidelberg cohort of the European Prospective Investigation into Cancer and Nutrition (EPIC-Heidelberg). *Am J Clin Nutr.* 2010 May;91(5):1348-58. Epub 2010 Mar 24.

Pearce KL, Clifton PM, Noakes M. Egg consumption as part of an energy-restricted high-protein diet improves blood lipid and blood glucose profiles in individuals with type 2 diabetes. *Br J Nutr.* 2010 Dec 7:1-8.

Pi-Sunyer X, The Medical Risks of Obesity. *Postgrad Med.* 2009 November; 121(6): 21–33.

Rees K, Guraewal S, Wong YL, Majanbu DL, Mavrodaris A, Stranges S, Kandala NB, Clarke A, Franco OH. Is vitamin K consumption associated with cardio-metabolic disorders? A systematic review. *Maturitas.* 2010 Oct;67(2):121-8. Epub 2010 Jun 17.

Roher B. Carbohydrate restriction fastest way to reduce triglycerides. Reported at The Liver Meeting 2010: American Association for the Study of Liver Diseases (AASLD) 61st Annual Meeting. Browning JD. http://www.medscape.com/viewarticle/732212

Strand RD. *Healthy for Life – Developing healthy lifestyles that have a side effect of permanent weight loss.* 2005. Rapid City SD: Real Life Press.

HERBS/SUPPLEMENTS

Autier P, Gandini S. Vitamin D supplementation and total mortality: a meta-analysis of randomized controlled trial. *Arch Internal Med,* 2007 Sep 10; 167(16): 1730-7.

Bernard K, Colon-Emeric C. Extraskeletal effects of vitamin D in older adults: cardiovascular disease, mortality, mood and cognition. *Am J Geriatr Pharmacother* 2010 Feb; 8(1): 4-33.

Bertone-Johnson ER. Vitamin D and breast cancer. *Ann Epidemiol* 2009 Jul; 19(7): 462-7.

Cannell JJ, Vieth R, Willett W, Zasloff M, Hathcock JN, White JH, Tanumihardjo SA, Larson-Meyer DE, Bischoff-Ferrari HA, Lamberg-Allardt CJ, Lappe JM, Norman AW, Zittermann A, Whiting SJ, Grant WB, Hollis BW, Biovannucci E. Cod liver oil, vitamin A toxicity, frequent respiratory infections, and the vitamin d deficiency epidemic. *Ann Otol Rhinol Laryngol.* 2008 Nov; 117(11): 864-70.

Freedman DM, Looker AC, Chang SC, Graubard BI. Prospective study of serum vitamin D and cancer mortality in the United States. *J Natl Cancer Inst.* 2007 Nov 7; 99(21): 1594-602.

Gaby, AR. 2011. *Nutritional Medicine.* Concord NH: Fritz Perlberg Publishing

Godel JC. Vitamin D supplementation: Recommended for Canadian mothers and infants. *Pediatr Child Health* 2007 September; 12 (7): 583-589.

Haskell CF, Scholey AB, Jackson PA, Elliott JM, Defeyter MA, Greer J, Robertson BC, Buchanan T, Tiplady B, Kennedy DO. Cognitive and mood effects in healthy children during 12 weeks' supplementation with multi-vitamin/minerals. *Br J Nutr.* 2008 Nov; 100(5): 1086-1096.

Huss M, Volp A, Stauss-Grabo M. Supplementation of polyunsaturated fatty acids, magnesium, and zinc in children seeking medical advice for attention-deficit/hyperactivity problems - an observational cohort study. *Lipids in Health and Disease* 2010; 9:105.

Institute of Medicine of the National Academies. *Dietary Reference for Calcium and Vitamin D Report.* November 20, 2010

Jacobs BP & Gundling K. *The ACP Evidence-Based Guide to Complementary and Alternative Medicine.* Philadelphia: ACP Press

LaValle J & Yale SL. *Cracking the Metabolic Code.* Laguna Beach CA: Basic Health Publications Inc.

Litonjua AA, Weiss ST. Is vitamin d deficiency to blame for the asthma epidemic. *J Allergy Clin Immunol,* 2007 Nov; 120(5): 1031-5

Office of Dietary Supplements, National Institute of Health. *Vitamin D.* Updated January 13, 2011

Sharief S, Jariwala S, Kumar J, Muntner P, Melamed M. Vitamin D levels and food and environmental allergies in the United States: Results from the National Health and Nutrition Examination Survey 2005-2006 *Journal of Allergy and Clinical Immunology,* published online 17 February 2011.

Sloan Kettering - www.mskcc.org/mskcc/html/11570.cfm

Smith PW. *What You Must Know About Vitamins, Minerals, Herbs & More ~ Choosing the Nutrients That Are Right For You.* Garden City Park NY: Square One Publishers.

Stargrove MB, Treasure T, McKee, DL. 2008. *Herb, Nutrient, and Drug Interactions – Clinical Implications and Therapeutic Strategies.* St Louis MO: Mosby Elsevier.

Wagner CL, Greer FR, et al. Prevention of rickets and vitamin d deficiency in infants, children, and adolescents. *Pediatrics* 2008; 122: 1142-1152.

HYGIENE HYPOTHESIS

Holt PG, van den Biggelaar AH. 99th Dahlem conference on infection, inflammation, and chronic inflammatory disorders: the role of infections in the allergy: atopic asthma as a paradigm. *Clin Exp Immunol.* 2010 Apr; 160(1)22-6

McDade TW, Rutherford J, Adair L, Kuzawa CW. Early origins of inflammation: microbial exposures in infancy predict lower levels of C-reactive protein in adulthood. *Proceedings of the Royal Society B (Biological Sciences),* November 17, 2009

Rook, GAW. Review Series on helminthes, immune modulators and the hygiene hypothesis; the broader implications of the hygiene hypothesis. *Immunology,* 2009. January; 126(1): 3-11.

Rautava S, Ruuskanen O, Ouwehand A, Salminen S, Isolauri E. The hygiene hypothesis of atopic disease - an extended version. *J Pediatr Gastroenterol Nutr.* 2004 Apr; 38(4) 378-388

Rook GA. Review series on helminths, immune modulation and hygiene hypothesis: The broader implications of the hygiene hypothesis. *Immunology,* 2009 January; 126(1):3-11.

POSTPARTUM DEPRESSION

Barclay L. Prevalence of self-reported postpartum depression symptoms ranges from 11.7% to 20.4%. *MMWR Mor Mortal Wkly Rep* 2008; 57(14): 361-366.

Bromley LA. Down and Out – How surviving postpartum depression made me a better doctor and person. *Can Fam Physician.* 2007 September: 53(9): 1527-1528

Sheeder JS, Kabir K, Stafford BS. Screening for postpartum depression at well-child visits: Is once enough during the first 6 months of life. *Pediatrics* 6 June 2009; 123(6): e982-e988

Sichel D & Driscoll JW. *Women's Moods – What every Woman must know about Hormones, the Brain, and Emotional Health.* (2000). New York NY: Quill

PREGNANCY

Bodnar LM, Catov JM, Dimhan HN, Holick MF, Powers RW, Roberts JM. Maternal vitamin d deficiency increases the risk of preeclampsia. *J Clin Endocrinol Metab.* 2007, Sep; 92(9): 3517-22

Bodnar LM, Krohn MA, Simhan HN. Maternal vitamin d deficiency is associated with bacterial vaginosis in the first trimester of pregnancy. *J Nutr.* 2009 Apr 8.

Boyles S. High doses of vitamin d may cut pregnancy risks. Reported at Pediatric Academic Societies annual meeting, British Columbia, May 1-4 2010. Wagner CL & Lawrence R. http://www.medscape.com/viewarticle/721294

Douglas, A. *The Mother of All Pregnancy Books – The Ultimate Guide to Conception, Birth and Everything in Between.* Hoboken NJ: Wiley Publishing Inc.

Gaby, AR. 2011. *Nutritional Medicine.* Concord NH: Fritz Perlberg Publishing

Javaid MK, Crozier SR, Harvey NC, Gale CR, Dennison EM, Boucher BJ, Arden NK, Godfrey KM, Cooper C. Maternal vitamin d status during pregnancy and childhood bone mass at age 9 years: a longitudinal study. *Lancet.* 2006 Jan 7; 367(9504): 36-43

Merewood A, Mehta SD, Chen TC, Bauchner H, Holick MF. Association between vitamin d deficiency and primary cesarean section. *J Endocrinol Metab.* 2009 Mar; 94(3): 940-9

Murkoff H & Mazel S. *What to Expect When You're Expecting.* New York NY: Workman Publishing Company.

Osaikhuwuamwan JA, Okpere EE, Okonkwo CA, Ande AB, Idogun ES. Plasma vitamin C levels and risk of preterm prelabour rupture of membranes. *Arch Gynecol Obstet* 2010 Nov 3.

Rauscher M. Prenatal vitamin d linked to kid's dental health. 2009 *Reuters.*

Stargrove MB, Treasure T, McKee, DL. 2008. *Herb, Nutrient, and Drug Interactions – Clinical Implications and Therapeutic Strategies.* St Louis MO: Mosby Elsevier.

Weed S. *The Wise Woman Herbal - Childbearing Years.* Woodstock NY: Ash Tree Publishing.

Zhang C, Qiu C, Hu FB, David RM, van Dam RM, Bralley A, Williams MA. Maternal plasma 25-hydroxyvitamin d concentrations and the risk for gestational diabetes mellitus.

PROBIOTICS

Barclay L. Clinical Report – A Review of Probiotics and Prebiotics for the American Academy of Pediatrics. *Pediatrics* November 29. 2010

Betsi GI, Papadavid E, Falagas ME. Probiotics for the treatment and prevent of atopic dermatitis: a review of the evidence from randomized controlled trials. *Am J Clin Dermatol* 2008; 9(2): 93-103

Gerasimov SV, Vasjuta VV, Myhovych OO, Bondarchuk LI. Probiotic supplement reduces atopic dermatitis in preschool children: a randomized, double-blind, placebo-controlled, clinical trial. *Am J Clin Dermatol,* 2010; 11(5):351-61.

Isolauri E, Kalliomaki M, Rautava S, Salminen S, Laitinen K. Obesity- extending the hygiene hypothesis. *Nestle Nutr Workshop Ser Pediatr Program* 2009; 64:75-85

Kim JY, Kwon JH, Ahn SH, Lee SI, Han YS, Choi YO, Lee SY, Ahn KM, Ji GE. Effect of probiotic mix in the primary prevention of eczema: a double-blind, randomized , placebo-controlled trial. *Pediatric Allergy and Immunology* October 2009; 9:2

Kligler B, Hanaway P, Cohrssen A. Probiotics in children. *Pediatric Clinics in N Am* 54 (2007) 949-967.

Savino F, Pelle E, Palumeri E, Oggero, R, Minier R, Margherita R Children's Hospital(Turin, Italy). *Lactobacillus reuteri* (American Type Culture Collection Strain 55730) Versus Simethicone in the Treatment of Infantile Colic: A Prospective Randomized Study. **Pediatrics** Vol. 119 No. 1 January 2007, pp. e124-e130

Thomas DW, Greer FR et al. Clinical report probiotics and prebiotics in pediatrics. *Pediatrics* Nov 29, 2010; DOI: 10.1542/peds.2010-2548.

Index

Acknowledgments

Thank you to . . .

My daughter, Stephanie Rose Noss, for opening my heart in ways I never imagined possible.

Tricia Reling, for your support, knowledge, and keeping me laughing out loud.

Sandy Ray, for standing by my side for over ten years, through thick and thin, and offering words of wisdom and compassion.

Terry Ball, for your words of wisdom, listening and listening, and making me laugh.

Clark and Karri Seger, for the love, laughter, and practical advice you give so freely.

Cheryl Seger Sellers, for being there during Stephanie's growing-up years.

Joann Fury and Jan Cotant, for your love, support, and advice on living life, being a parent, and the joys of being a grandparent.

Lyn Benke, who taught Stephanie and me how to have fun baking Christmas cookies, and a whole bunch of other stuff.

Sahar Swidan, for sharing her incredible knowledge regarding supplements for children and adults, for introducing me to the American Academy of Anti-Aging Medicine and the Fellowship program and best of all her unique blend of intelligence and humor.

Mary Jo Zazueta, my editor, for your patience and kindness in taking so much information and consolidating it into what is written within these pages

The women in my life, who have guided me, loved me, supported me, picked me up, brushed me off, and sent me back into the game of life. Thank you, I have been blessed. It has taken a village.

My husband, Bill Baughman. There are not enough words to express how much I love you and appreciate your love and support. Thank you for being in my life.